About the author

Clare Byam-Cook trained as a nurse at Westminster Hospital and qualified in 1976. After going on to do a midwifery course at Pembury Hospital in Kent and qualifying as a midwife in 1979, she then worked for four years at Queen Charlotte's Hospital in London until the birth of her first baby. In 1989 Clare was approached by antenatal teacher Christine Hill to join Hill's Chiswick practice as her breast-feeding specialist and she has been there ever since.

During her years working with Christine Hill, Clare has gained invaluable experience in everything to do with breast-feeding, bottle-feeding, crying babies (and crying mothers!), and everything else associated with the day-to-day care of newborn babies. In addition to teaching at the antenatal classes, she makes home visits to any mother who asks for her help, and says she has learnt more about babies and feeding problems from doing these home visits than in all her years spent working as a hospital midwife.

Clare has gained a reputation for being able to solve almost any breastfeeding problem and all her clients come to her by word-of-mouth referral from their friends, GPs, obstetricians, paediatricians, midwives and health visitors. Clare has never advertised her services and says that when the referrals dry up she knows it will be time for her to retire!

Clare feels that there is no better experience to be acquired than by being in a position to see the same problems time and time again. As a result, most of the advice she gives in this book is based on the knowledge she has gained during the many years she has been doing these home visits. It is not based solely on textbook theories.

In praise of Clare and her advice

'Whenever I refer patients to Clare I am confident that, if the problem can be solved, she will solve it. Her expertise and calm, confident manner has provided help and reassurance to countless mothers over the years.'

Dr Tim Evans (Royal Physician)

'With Mia I had real problems getting her to latch on and was close to giving up when I got advice from Clare. I just can't praise her enough – she has a really straightforward way of describing the latching-on technique and has managed to get mothers breast-feeding when they really thought they would never get it.'

Kate Winslet

'This book should be handed out with the first contraction. Clare is a true "baby whisperer" who will save you and your baby hours of torment. Her kind, commonsense and amazingly informed advice was as essential to me as breastpads and chocolate. Buy this book!'

Kate Beckinsale

'I booked Clare to come round the day my fourth child was born, and the breast-feeding has, for the first time, worked from the first day.'

Emma Freud

'Breast-feeding is one of those things you go through life assuming to be natural and easy, but when I was pregnant I began to hear lots of horror stories about bleeding nipples and awful pain. So I booked Clare to come and see me by way of a pre-emptive strike. It was fantastic. She showed me how to place the baby at the right level using a pillow and pretty early on I was able to feed him, hands-free.'

Helena Bonham Carter

'When I read Clare's book I realised how much I had to learn, and how much could so easily go wrong. The hour or so I spent with her was one of the most valuable in my "motherhood" preparation. I always thought that breast-feeding would be a chore but I have to say it is one of the highlights of my day.'

Gabby Logan

'Despite being a professional working with children I soon realised that at a personal level common sense can go out of the window. As an uncle and more recently a father I have very gratefully acepted Clare's straight-talking, no-nonsense approach. Not only do I now have a niece and son who eat and consequently sleep better but Clare's invaluable help has resulted in four happier parents as well.'

Atul J Sabhawal, Consultant Paediatric Surgeon

clare byam-cook

what to expect when you're breast-feeding... and what if you can't?

Vermilion
LONDON

5 7 9 10 8 6 4

First published in the United Kingdom in 2001 by Vermilion

This edition published in the United Kingdom in 2006
by Vermilion, an imprint of Ebury Publishing
Random House UK Ltd.
Random House
20 Vauxhall Bridge Road
London SW1V 2SA

Random House Australia (Pty) Limited
20 Alfred Street, Milsons Point, Sydney,
New South Wales, 2061, Australia

Random House New Zealand Limited
18 Poland Road, Glenfield,
Auckland 10, New Zealand

Random House (Pty) Limited
Isle of Houghton, Corner of Boundary Road & Carse O'Gowrie,
Houghton, 2198, South Africa

Random House Publishers India Private Limited
301 World Trade Tower, Hotel Intercontinental Grand Complex,
Barakhamba Lane, New Delhi 110 001, India

Random House UK Limited Reg. No. 954009
www.randomhouse.co.uk

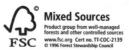

Mixed Sources
Product group from well-managed
forests and other controlled sources
www.fsc.org Cert no. TT-COC-2139
© 1996 Forest Stewardship Council

A CIP catalogue record is available for this book from the British Library.

ISBN: 9780091906962

Typeset by SX Composing DTP, Rayleigh, Essex
Printed and bound in Great Britain
by Mackays of Chatham plc, Chatham, Kent

Please note that conversions to imperial weights and measures are suitable equivalents and not exact.

The information given in this book should not be treated as a substitute for qualified medical advice; always consult a medical practitioner. Neither the author nor the publisher can be held responsible for any loss or claim arising out of the use, or misuse, of the suggestions made or the failure to take medical advice.

Contents

Acknowledgements   ix
Author's note   xi
Introduction   1

1   Preparing for breast-feeding   5
Equipment   5
Preparing the nipples   8
Diet   9
Fluid intake   12

2   How breast-feeding works   13
Breast size and milk production   14
How breasts produce milk   14
Supply and demand   16
The let-down reflex   17
Foremilk and hindmilk   18
One breast or two?   19
Afterpains when feeding   21

3   How to do a breast-feed   23
The ideal breast-feeding position   24
Doing a breast-feed   25
Winding   35
Swaddling   38
Settling your baby after feeds   40
Different feeding positions   41

4   The first few days   47
When your baby is born   47
The first 24 hours   47
Before your milk comes in   55
When your milk comes in   57

5   Coming home from hospital   61
Rest   61
Visitors   62

Cot death – safety for baby 62
Where your baby should sleep 63
Room temperature 65
Help in the home 66
Maternity nurses 67
Doulas 69
District midwives 69
Health visitor 70

6 General feeding advice 71
Feeding twins 71
Drugs and breast-feeding 74
Breast surgery 74
Weight gain 75
How much milk does your baby need? 77
What about extra water? 78
How long should a feed last? 78
Feeding on demand 80
Feeding on a strict four-hourly schedule 83
Settling into a routine 84
Waking at 10pm? 86
Night feeds 86
Dummies 87
Expressing milk 89
Introducing a bottle 94
Ideal length of time to breast-feed 95
Weaning from breast to bottle 96
Breast-feeding and the working mother 99

7 Common feeding problems for mothers 101
Inverted nipples 101
Baby can't latch on 102
Sore nipples 107
Primary engorgement 113
Vascular engorgement 117
Blocked milk ducts 118
Mastitis 119
Breast abscess 121
Too much milk 122
Milk flow is too fast 123

Not enough breast milk 125
Growth spurts 129
Baby 'fussing' at the breast 130
Baby can't or won't suck efficiently 131
The ill mother 133

8   Common feeding problems for baby 135
Jaundice 135
The sleepy baby 137
The unsettled baby 137
Poor weight gain 141
Milk allergy/food intolerance 143
Colic 144
Evening colic/evening fretting 148
Gastro-oesophageal reflux 148
Constipation 153
Thrush 153
Dehydration 155
Refusing bottles 156
Baby in special care baby unit 161

9   Bottle-feeding 163
Equipment 163
Sterilising 165
Different types of formula milk 168
Making up the feeds 169
Giving the feed 171
Baby bottle tooth decay 173
Excessive weight gain 173
Poor weight gain (when bottle-feeding) 174

10   Other issues 177
Tongue-tie 177
White nipple 178
Cranial osteopathy 178
Starting solids 180
How to get your baby to sleep through the night 182

Final note 185

Useful information and contacts 187
Index 189

Acknowledgements

My thanks to . . .

My son Richard, without whose help this book would never have been written. Richard taught me from scratch how to use a computer and then put up with my endless cries for help every time I couldn't make it do what I wanted. How nice that he has graduated from being a difficult baby (see page 147) into such a helpful adult!

My daughter Susan, who dealt with my computer disasters whenever Richard was unavailable. She too has turned into a pretty useful daughter!

My husband David, who has provided support and encouragement throughout all my ventures. In particular I want to thank him for being prepared to listen to absolutely endless (and for him, extremely boring!) discussions on all aspects of this book – not many men would be so tolerant.

Christine Hill, for giving me so much help in the writing of this book. Her advice and expertise has been invaluable.

And, finally, I would like to thank all the doctors, paediatricians and new mothers who took the time to read the manuscript and give me their constructive feedback.

Author's note

The main purpose in writing this book is to help mothers who are experiencing breast-feeding problems. These are the women I see day in, day out (mothers without problems rarely ring me!) and who I feel will benefit most from reading it. I have therefore written the book as a step-by-step problem-solving guide, on the premise that it will mainly be read by mothers who are having problems, rather than those who are not. However, there will undoubtedly be others who will want to read it in order to help them avoid problems arising in the first place.

I'm assuming that many women will not want to read this book from cover to cover before their baby is born, but will instead only refer to it if they are actually having a feeding problem. For this reason, I have tried to cover each problem in its entirety without having too many cross-references. As a result, some of my advice is repeated several times throughout.

To avoid confusion between the mother who is female and her baby who could be either sex, I have referred to the baby throughout as being male.

Finally, for ease of writing, and to avoid endless references to the father of the baby as 'partner, other half or husband', I have decided to opt for 'husband'. This does not mean that I assume everyone is married.

Introduction

The health benefits associated with breast-feeding are so numerous that every mother really does owe it to her baby at least to attempt to breast-feed. Although it will not *guarantee* your baby perfect health for the rest of his life, there is plenty of evidence to show that he will benefit hugely if you can manage to breast-feed him for the first six months. A breast-fed baby is less likely to suffer from gastro-enteritis, ear and urinary tract infections, allergies, eczema, diabetes, heart disease and obesity. He will also be protected from diseases to which his mother has built up an immunity.

Many mothers sail through breast-feeding from the word go. They find it all blissfully easy and simply can't understand how anyone could have a problem with such a 'natural' aspect of mothering. But they are the lucky ones!

The reality is that breast-feeding is not nearly as easy as everyone makes out and the sad fact is that almost 50 per cent of mothers give up breast-feeding within the first six weeks because they find it too difficult or painful. Most mothers assume that it will be wonderful, easy and natural, and it comes as quite a shock when they experience problems – they then feel totally inadequate and distraught if they can't resolve these problems. For these mothers I would like to point out that breast-feeding may well be natural, but it is still a skill that has to be learned and many women will only be successful if they get proper, skilled help from the outset. Unfortunately, this help is not always available, and many experience problems that result in them not only giving up breast-feeding, but then blaming themselves for their so-called 'failure'. I feel very strongly that a mother should **not** feel a failure if she is finding breast-feeding difficult and is not being helped by any of the health professionals – if we, the 'experts', can't offer a solution to her problems, it is quite wrong for the mother to feel the failure. *We* are the failure!

Having said this, I do firmly believe that not all women can breast-feed (even given expert help) as our bodies are not perfect and do not always work as well as they should. Breasts are like any other part of our body, and nature can no more guarantee that they will always work perfectly than it can guarantee everyone will have, for example, perfect eyesight. And yet a person suffering from poor eyesight is given sympathy and would not be told that if she tried harder her eyes would work better! It therefore follows that, however correctly some mothers breast-feed, some will find that their breasts let them down and that there is absolutely nothing that they (or anyone else) can do to improve matters.

I would like to stress that for the vast majority of mothers, problems normally only occur when they are breast-feeding incorrectly and that, given the right help and advice, almost every problem can be resolved.

The most common breast-feeding problems experienced by many mothers are:

- an inability to latch the baby on the breast
- sore nipples
- engorged breasts
- mastitis
- not having enough milk.

Most mothers experiencing these problems are told: 'Your breast is too big', 'Your baby's mouth is too small', 'Sore nipples are part and parcel of breast-feeding (and will get better given time)', 'It's just bad luck', etc., etc. When I visit these mothers, I am nearly always able to prove to them that none of these is the case. It normally takes me about 30 seconds to get a baby on the breast and I would usually expect sore nipples to heal up within 24 hours or so of my visit. Similarly, engorged breasts will usually feel more comfortable within minutes of the baby sucking correctly on the breast and mastitis rarely recurs once I have shown a mother how to position her baby on the breast.

Whenever I am consulted by a mother, I nearly always go through the same procedure:

- I ask her to show me what she *has* been doing
- I then show her what she *should* be doing
- I then get the mother to do whatever I have just shown her so that we are both sure that she will be able to manage on her own when I am not there to help her.

I have always found this to be the best approach because, doing it like this, we can both see the results of my help. For example, if a mother rings me to say that she can't get her baby to latch on the breast, she might think it's just good luck if her baby then latches on when I visit a few hours later. But if she fails to get her baby on the breast while I am watching her, and I then have no trouble putting the baby on the breast a few minutes later, she'll find it much easier to see that this is down to technique rather than luck! In the same way, a mother with agonisingly sore nipples can feel the pain subside as soon as I move the baby to the correct position.

Virtually every mother I see with feeding problems has been to antenatal classes (including my own!), has read many books on breast-feeding and yet still finds breast-feeding difficult. This is because what seems logical and easy before the baby is born becomes a totally different matter when the mother is trying to cope with a wriggling, crying and hungry baby. It is for these women that I have written this book, in the hope that my advice will help them in their hour of need.

If, however . . .

- the book doesn't help you (and nor does anyone else)
- everything is going horribly wrong and you and your baby are permanently in tears
- your husband has started finding excuses to stay away from home or
- you are hating every second of breast-feeding,

. . . it is probably better to give up the whole idea and restore peace and calm to the household – even if it means giving a bottle! Do remember, though, that most problems are very temporary and, having given one or two bottle feeds, it may still be worth per-severing with breast-feeding for a few more days to see whether things get better. If things do improve, then you will have many months ahead of you to enjoy it, and if they don't, at least you will always know that you gave it your best effort. Whatever the outcome, the most important thing is that you and your baby are happy and thriving and that he gets enough milk.

1 Preparing for breast-feeding

One of the joys of breast-feeding is that you will need very little equipment. In fact, in theory you shouldn't need any at all as you already possess the most important equipment that you will need – your breasts! However, in reality most mothers will buy maternity bras, breast pads, etc., as these, while not essential, will certainly make breast-feeding more comfortable. I would also recommend that all breast-feeding mothers have some bottle-feeding equipment in their house for use in an emergency. I don't wish to frighten breast-feeding mothers by talking about emergencies, but an occasion may arise when they will be very glad if they have a bottle to hand. Such occasions are mentioned later on in the chapters covering breast-feeding problems. In any event it is essential that a breast-fed baby learns to take some feeds from a bottle: unless a breast-fed baby is given the occasional bottle-feed (of expressed breast milk) there is a risk that he will refuse point-blank to take a bottle when, for example, you have to go back to work.

Equipment
Breast-feeding does not require nearly as much equipment as bottle-feeding, as it is normally possible to make do with things that you already have in the kitchen. For example, bottles can be sterilised in any non-metallic container (such as an old, clean ice-cream tub) using a sterilising fluid, or they can be boiled in a saucepan, thus making it unnecessary to purchase a sterilising unit. It is best to avoid buying anything that is not completely essential because your house has no doubt already become cluttered with an enormous amount of baby paraphernalia and the last thing you want to do is to add to it.

You will need:

- a box of disposable breast pads or a minimum of 18 washable ones
- at least three well-fitting maternity bras
- a tube of nipple cream, e.g. Lansinoh, Kamillosan or Calendula
- at least one bottle and teat
- a bottle brush
- a steam steriliser, or a small bottle of sterilising fluid/packet of sterilising tablets (see pages 165–168).

Breast pads

Breast pads are worn inside the bra to prevent milk from leaking onto your bra and/or clothes. There are two types: washable and disposable. The washable variety are more economical and are environmentally friendly, but you may prefer the convenience of the disposable type.

Maternity bras

Maternity bras will provide the extra support you need when breast-feeding. They have the advantage of having zip- or hook-fastened openings on the cups, so that you can feed your baby without having to undo your bra at the back.

Nipple creams

I cannot stress enough that the main cause of sore nipples is incorrect latching of the baby to the breast – if your baby latches correctly from the outset you are extremely unlikely to suffer any pain. Nonetheless, a good nipple cream will usually aid healing if a mother does develop sore nipples, and may also provide some protection for women with delicate nipples who are particularly vulnerable to this problem. You should use a nipple cream in much the same way as you would a sun cream – frequently at first, then tailing off gradually. I suggest that you start by using it at every feed and then gradually reduce the frequency until you feel able to stop it altogether.

Note: A mother with sensitive skin may find that she reacts badly to certain nipple creams, in which case the cream will do more harm than good.

You may also need:

- a breast pump
- two nipple shields
- two breast shells (if your breasts leak a lot of milk in between feeds)
- a small carton of ready-made formula milk (as a back-up if you are temporarily unable to breast-feed).

Breast pumps

Most women won't need a breast pump, but many find it extremely useful, either for convenience, or during temporary breast-feeding problems such as sore nipples or engorged breasts. Breast pumps vary enormously in price, size and ease of assembly and operation, with the more expensive ones tending to be quieter and more efficient than the cheaper ones. As a general rule, you will find that the better your milk flows, the easier it is to express and the less sophisticated your breast pump needs to be. Given the wide choice available, I recommend that you decide in advance which would best suit your needs (and bank balance!) so that you are not rushed into making a decision after your baby is born. There are two main types: manual and electric/battery operated.

Manual: These pumps are widely available and are operated entirely by hand, using suction to extract the milk. The advantage of a manual pump is that it is very portable, is cheaper than an electric pump and works well if you have a good flow of milk. However, if your milk supply is low (and you are expressing to try and boost it), or if your milk flows very slowly, you may find a manual breast pump fairly ineffective and tiring to use, and would do better to try an electric pump.

Electric/battery-operated: These can be bought from most large chemists and department stores, or through mail order catalogues. Electric pumps are almost as small and portable as a manual pump but are usually more effective and are well worth buying if you are planning (or need) to express on a regular basis. You will also have the choice between buying a single or double pump – the double pumps are, of course, generally more expensive than a single pump but have the advantage of being quicker to use as you can express simultaneously from both breasts.

Note: Some mothers choose to rent a breast pump, but generally it makes more sense to buy your own, particularly if you are planning to have more than one baby.

Nipple shields

You will only need these if you are having a breast-feeding problem, such as sore nipples or difficulty in latching your baby on. There are many types on the market and most of them work well, provided the mother has a fast flow of milk (see page 109). However, most of the shields available in the shops are fairly large in size and I find that the majority of babies suck more effectively when using a smaller shield, made by Medela. The Medela shields are also very well designed, with a cut-away section that allows the baby's nose to touch and smell the breast as he feeds. Medela products are available in some shops and also through mail order (see Useful information and contacts, page 187).

Breast shells

A breast shell is a small plastic device that fits over your nipple and is held in place by your bra. It can be used to collect milk if your breasts leak a lot in between feed times, or if you leak from one breast while the baby is feeding from the other. Any milk that is collected can then be stored in the fridge, or frozen for use at a later date.

All the above can be bought from most chemists, specialist baby shops and the Baby section in big department stores. A good chemist will normally get in for you anything they do not already have in stock.

Preparing the nipples

Virtually every mother seems to live in fear of getting sore nipples as soon as she starts breast-feeding and wants to know whether there is anything she can do in advance to stop this happening. It might help to rub your nipples with a dry towel after a bath during the last month of pregnancy to toughen them up a bit, or to use nipple cream right from the very first feed, but neither of these should really be necessary. If your nipples do become sore when you start breast-feeding it is more likely to be due to your baby latching on incorrectly than as a result of having delicate, unprepared nipples. By far the best way to prevent sore nipples is to make sure that when your baby is born he latches on correctly, right from the very first feed.

Nipple creams used to be very popular and were recommended as an essential part of breast-feeding equipment. Some hospitals are still in favour of them, while others are against, feeling that they contribute nothing when it comes to preventing or healing sore nipples.

Instead of nipple cream, they may suggest that you rub a little bit of your own breast milk on to your nipple at the end of each feed, or that you use their own tried-and-tested remedy such as grated raw carrot. If you get sore nipples there is no harm in trying anything that might help to speed up the healing process. However, if you do decide to use a nipple cream, make sure that you only use one that is designed to be safe to go into the mouth of a newborn baby. Be sure to choose one that's suitable for breast-feeding mothers and follow the instructions on the packet.

Note: Many of my clients tell me that they have heard that putting white spirit on their nipples will help to toughen them up. I don't know where this idea came from but it is not something that I would recommend!

Diet

During pregnancy
During pregnancy it is important to eat a good healthy diet, both for the sake of your unborn baby and in preparation for breast-feeding. Some foods may be potentially harmful to the baby and should therefore be avoided, whilst other foods will have a beneficial effect on him. You should also plan to increase your calorie intake by approximately 200–300 calories a day – many more than this may cause you to put on too much weight and much fewer could deprive your growing baby of the extra nutrients he needs.

Try to eat a healthy, well-balanced diet, and in particular:

- Help your baby to lay down calcium in his bones by eating dairy products, meat, green vegetables, nuts, seeds, pulses and beans.
- Help yourself by eating iron-rich foods such as meat, spinach, lentils, green vegetables and salad. You can also take iron supplements.

Avoid:

- Any food containing raw eggs (e.g. mousses and mayonnaise) because of the risk of salmonella.
- All soft and blue-veined cheese, and any other unpasteurised dairy products. These may contain listeria bacteria which are harmful to the unborn baby.
- Raw or under-cooked meat (e.g. pâté or pork) as these may contain a parasite which can cause Toxoplasmosis. This may result in miscarriage, premature birth or damage to the baby.
- All supplements containing vitamin A, and any food (especially liver) which contains high levels of vitamin A. Large quantities of vitamin A can cause birth defects.
- Peanuts and peanut products (e.g. unrefined groundnut oil) if you have a family history of allergies. These may trigger a nut allergy in your baby.

Although most health professionals are in full agreement on the subject of diet during pregnancy, there seems to be no such consensus of opinion on the subject of alcohol. Some studies state that alcohol consumed in *small* amounts (2–4 units a week) will cause no harm, while others state than any alcohol at all poses an unacceptable risk to the baby. On the basis of this, it is clearly best to consume as little alcohol as possible both during pregnancy and when breast-feeding.

When breast-feeding

While you are breast-feeding you will still need to eat healthily, as the food you eat will be used partly to provide energy for you and partly to make milk for your baby. There are no hard-and-fast rules about how much you should eat, but you should expect to eat and drink slightly more than usual and, in particular, make sure that you eat on a regular basis. This doesn't mean that you'll have to spend hours preparing meals (sandwiches, etc., are fine), but you should ideally have at least one hot meal a day. Don't worry about putting on weight because a lot of the calories you'll be consuming will be used up in producing milk for the baby. As a general rule, it's best to be guided by hunger and your milk supply, i.e. if your milk supply is low, eat more and make sure that you are not skipping meals because you are too tired or too busy to eat.

Contrary to what some mothers think, you can eat pretty much whatever you like, as there are no foods that definitely have to be avoided when you are breast-feeding. However, there are certain foods that are likely either to affect your baby's digestion, or to change the flavour of your milk and are therefore probably best avoided. Use the following information as a guide:

- You can now eat soft and blue-veined cheeses, pâté and liver as these should not affect your baby via the breast milk.
- For your own health, you should still be wary of potentially risky foods such as raw eggs.
- Peanut products should still be avoided if you have a strong family history of allergies.
- Your baby might be affected if you eat garlic, hot spicy foods such as curries, or citrus fruits (if eaten in excess). If any of these happen to be your favourites there's no harm in experimenting to see if your baby objects to them. You may find that they have no effect on him at all, especially if they are foods that you have been eating regularly throughout your pregnancy.
- No one knows exactly how long it takes for the milk supply to be affected by food or drink, but it will probably take at least four hours for it to enter the milk. If your baby does become very unsettled after you have eaten something unusual, avoid that food for a week or two, then try eating it again to see if he reacts in the same way. If he does, you will know that *your* baby doesn't like you eating that particular food – but this doesn't mean that you need to ring up all your friends and warn them not to eat it either!
- If you do eat something that doesn't agree with your baby, the most common reaction you can expect is for him to become more unsettled and/or windy or to suffer from mild diarrhoea. This will not do him any harm although it won't be much fun for either of you while it lasts. You may also find that he fusses a lot at the breast or feeds less well if you have eaten something, such as garlic, that affects the taste of the milk.
- Milk and dairy products provide essential calcium for you and your baby, so if you think your baby is reacting to them badly don't cut them out of your diet without first seeking medical advice.

Fluid intake

Mothers are usually advised to drink extra fluids when they are breast-feeding, but most find that thirst automatically makes them drink more than they normally would anyway. If your milk supply is good, whatever you are drinking is probably enough, but if it's low and you have dark-coloured urine, you should drink more.

If you are like me and find it hard to drink plenty of water, you may find it helpful to fill at least one large jug with water each morning and try to finish it by the end of the day. I say this because I know from experience that many women think they are drinking more water than they actually are, so using a jug will be a good way to keep track.

The best fluids to drink are water and milk, but tea and coffee are fine, as long as you don't drink them to excess – too much caffeine can make both you and your baby a bit jittery. Alcohol does go through to the breast milk so although the occasional drink is unlikely to do either of you any harm, the less you drink the better. Fizzy drinks are best avoided as they will tend to give your baby indigestion.

Note: If your milk supply is low, there is an old wives' tale that suggests drinking Guinness will help you to make more milk. I have to say that I have not found much evidence to support this theory, but in any event I would not recommend drinking alcohol as a way to boost milk production.

2 How breast-feeding works

When breast-feeding goes well (as it does for many, many women), a mother does not need to know how or why it works, and will find it extremely easy, enjoyable and satisfying. This is what should happen:

- Your baby wakes up hungry.
- You put him to the breast for a feed.
- He sucks at the breast until he has had enough milk, at which point he falls fast asleep.
- He sleeps soundly until he is hungry and wants another feed (three to four hours later).
- You put him back to the breast and he has another feed. He then goes to sleep and the cycle starts all over again.

When breast-feeding works like this, the mother has no reason to worry about how much milk her baby needs, how much he is getting, or how much she is producing. All she knows is that whenever her baby is hungry she can put him to the breast and that there will be enough milk for him. Her baby will be calm and content and will be gaining the right amount of weight. She will have no bottles to sterilise, no feeds to make up and no equipment to take with her when she goes out. This is what breast-feeding is all about and this is how it should be for all mothers.

Unfortunately, it is not always this easy, which is why so many books have been written on the subject! But understanding how breast-feeding works will help you to know what to do when things go wrong and, better still, will help you to prevent them from going wrong in the first place.

Breast size and milk production

Most women find that their breasts get bigger when they are pregnant. Although the increase in size can vary considerably from one woman to another, this size variation doesn't seem to have any bearing on how much milk the breasts produce when the baby is born. Contrary to popular opinion, breast size does not affect milk production. If you have breasts hanging down to your knees, you should not be complacent and think that you will sail through breast-feeding; neither should you assume that, if all you have are two little mole hills sitting on your chest wall, you will be unable to breast-feed!

The reason breast size does not affect milk production is because large breasts are large purely because they have more fatty tissue in them than small breasts, not because they have more milk-producing cells. Nonetheless, I continue to be amazed by how much milk can come out of the tiniest breasts, and equally surprised by how inefficient some enormous breasts prove to be. I find it very noticeable that while some mothers produce masses of milk right from the word go, other mothers really struggle to produce enough and this seems to bear absolutely no relation to the size of their breasts. As there is no way of telling in advance how effective breasts will be when it comes to milk production, each mother has to wait until her baby is born to see whether nature has been kind to her!

How breasts produce milk

Milk is made in the breasts by milk-producing cells and is then stored in small bunches of milk sacs, which are distributed all over the breast (see opposite). Tiny ducts from these milk sacs lead down to a collecting area behind the nipple and from here the milk is squirted into the baby's mouth every time he sucks. In order for him to get this milk easily, he needs to be latched on in such a way that his jaws can reach well beyond the nipple to this collecting area. This usually means that he will need to take the whole nipple and a large part of the areola (the brown area around the nipple) into his mouth.

Colostrum

Towards the end of pregnancy the breasts start producing a small amount of milk in readiness for the birth of the baby, so that some milk will be there for him if he is born before his due date. This early

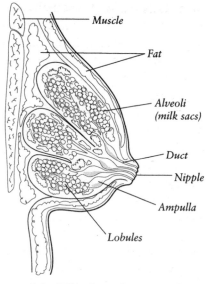

Muscle

Fat

Alveoli
(milk sacs)

Duct

Nipple

Ampulla

Lobules

A lactating breast

milk is called colostrum and is the milk that your baby will have for the first three or four days before your full milk comes in.

Although there is not much of this colostrum, it is full of goodness and antibodies and is nearly always enough for your baby. In fact, it's so good for him that you will have got him off to a really good start by giving him this, even if you only manage to breast-feed for these first few days.

Note: The antibodies in the colostrum will only provide your baby with protection to resist infections to which *you* have built up an immunity. This means that breast-feeding will not protect him from minor illnesses such as coughs and colds, so you shouldn't feel let down if your baby does get a cold (or any other such illness) while you are still breast-feeding.

Milk

Your milk won't come in until the levels of progesterone and oestrogen fall (this starts to happen as soon as your placenta is delivered), allowing prolactin levels to rise enough to stimulate the milk-producing cells to start producing milk. This can take anything from two to four days, which explains why some mothers have to wait longer than others. A small number of mothers might find that their milk doesn't come in until Day 5. If this happens to you, you may need to give your baby some formula milk to tide him over. This is unlikely to affect your breast-feeding, but nonetheless you should only offer him formula at this point on the advice of a paediatrician or midwife if their opinion is that your baby clearly needs more milk than your breasts are providing.

You will know when your milk has come in because your breasts will become firmer and a lot fuller and the colour of the milk will change from the yellowish consistency of colostrum to a watery milky colour.

As it is the delivery of your placenta that alters your hormonal balance and gets milk production under way, the type of delivery you have will not affect how soon your milk comes in. Even if you cannot feed at all for the first few days, it will still come in. However, once it does, you will need to feed every few hours throughout the day *and* night in order to keep your breasts stimulated enough to match your baby's milk requirements.

Note: Increasingly my clients say they are being told that having a Caesarian section will delay their milk coming in. I have seen no evidence of this, but whether or not it's true, there is nothing you can do about it, so there is no point worrying about it.

Supply and demand

Breast milk is produced on a supply-and-demand basis, which means the breasts will supply whatever the baby demands and the more he demands, the more they will supply. Initially they will normally produce enough milk for your baby, regardless of how big or hungry he is, and they will make more as he gets older without your even being aware of it. You will never know for sure how much milk your breasts are producing, or how much your baby is taking from them, but it will be obvious that he is getting enough if he is sleeping well and gaining weight.

As breasts can't see or hear what is going on, they work by reacting to whatever happens to them. They know that whenever they get emptied they must fill up again and that the more milk that is extracted from them, the more they must produce. When the baby stops sucking at the end of a feed this tells the breasts that the baby has had enough, and gives them the message that they will need to produce approximately the same amount at the next feed. When he comes back to the breast for the next feed, the second message they will get is that the amount of milk they produced at the previous feed was enough to keep him satisfied for the length of time between the two feeds. It is the combination of these two messages that tell the breasts whether they are producing too much or too little milk, or getting it exactly right.

As long as you continue to feed your baby whenever he is hungry (rather than making him stick to a strict and inflexible feeding schedule) your breasts will normally increase or decrease the amount of milk they are producing to keep in step with his requirements. In other words, if your breasts find that they are producing much more milk than your baby needs, they will gradually cut back on production and if they are producing too little, they will make more.

A breast-fed baby will normally take varying amounts of milk at each feed, with the amount sometimes differing by several ounces. To allow for this, efficient breasts will normally make sure that there is always some left over at the end of each feed to allow for the occasions when he might want a slightly bigger feed than usual. They will not assume that they are producing too much milk if a small amount is left over and, by the same token, they will not immediately double production if your baby occasionally has a large feed.

The let-down reflex

This is the mechanism that controls the flow of milk from the breasts, releasing the milk when the baby sucks and holding it in when he doesn't. The reason you need to know about it is because it is the let-down reflex that affects how fast the milk flows, and which in turn dictates how long your baby will need to suck in order to empty your breast.

The rate of milk flow varies enormously from mother to mother, with some having a very fast let-down reflex, others having a very slow let-down and the majority having a normal or average one. A mother has no control over her let-down reflex and it is very much the luck of the draw as to how fast or slow it is, although it does sometimes seem to slow down if a mother is very tense and anxious.

You'll find it is very easy to tell if you have a fast let-down reflex as you will see milk dripping or spurting from your breasts before you can even latch your baby on and you will then hear him gulping and swallowing and sometimes choking on the milk as he feeds. You will also find that after as little as ten minutes' sucking, he may have had enough milk and won't want to feed any more. The advantage of a fast let-down reflex is that feeding times are very short, but the disadvantage is that the baby often takes in a lot of air and as a result may take a long time to wind and settle. In addition, some babies may be unable to cope if the milk flow is much too fast, and can become panicky and start refusing to suck at the breast. Using a nipple shield (see page 109) can usually cure this problem.

It is harder to distinguish between average and slow let-down reflexes as these do not show such obvious physical signs. With an average let-down, it will take your baby about 20 minutes to get enough milk, whereas it can take anything from 25 minutes to an hour if you have a slower let-down. You may find it helpful to time each feed and keep notes so that you can see approximately how long your feeds last and see whether this bears any relation to how long your baby sleeps after each feed.

As a general rule, most mothers find that their milk tends to flow at a fairly similar speed throughout the feed (fast, normal or slow, depending on their let-down reflex) until the point when the breast is nearly empty, when it will usually start to slow down. However, a breast will sometimes release the milk in 'waves', resulting in a period of time when the baby will get no milk (however hard he sucks) until the next wave of milk is let down. If there is too long a delay (more than three or four minutes) a baby will often become impatient and will show this by crying and fussing, and generally not feeding well. If this seems to be happening, you should try moving him onto the other breast, even if he hasn't been sucking for very long and is unlikely to have completely emptied the first breast – you can always bring him back to this later on in the feed. Sometimes you will find that you need to keep moving your baby from breast to breast as this will be the only way to give him a continuous flow of milk.

Foremilk and hindmilk

There is a lot of confusion and misunderstanding about the composition of breast milk, with the result that many mothers are given both misleading and incorrect advice on the subject. The general conception seems to be that breasts produce two *totally* different kinds of milk – the foremilk, which comes out first, and then the hindmilk, which is sitting right at the back like a little pot of liquid gold and which will only be reached if the breast is *completely* emptied. With this in mind, mothers are told any of the following:

● You should only use one breast per feed (to ensure that the

hindmilk is reached).
- You must empty one breast before you swap to the other.
- It will take a baby precisely 20 minutes to reach the hindmilk – or 30 or 40 minutes, depending on the view of the person relaying this information!

In fact, what actually happens is that the composition of breast milk changes *gradually* as a baby feeds. This means that he will start off with plenty of thirst-quenching and low-calorie foremilk and, as the milk flow slows down, the fat and calorie content will rise – this is the hindmilk.

The amount of time it takes for a baby to reach this hindmilk will vary enormously from woman to woman – it will depend upon the speed of the mother's let-down reflex and upon how well the baby is positioned at her breast. It is therefore totally incorrect to dictate exactly how long a baby needs to feed in order to reach this hindmilk, or to state that a breast must be *completely* empty before the second breast is offered.

The best way to find out whether your baby is getting the right mix of foremilk and hindmilk is to see how long he settles in between feeds, how content he is and whether he is gaining the right amount of weight. If his weight gain is good you can be fairly sure he is getting the correct proportion of foremilk and hindmilk, but if he appears unsettled and hungry and his weight gain is poor you may need to adjust the way you are feeding. You can do this by allowing him to spend longer sucking on the first breast before you go on to the second. (See One breast or two?, below.)

Note: There is a school of thought that suggests that breasts are capable of working out how to balance the proportion of foremilk and hindmilk so that the baby always gets the correct mixture. I tend to agree with this as I find that most babies thrive perfectly well when using both breasts at every feed. Presumably this is because once the breasts know how much milk the baby is taking out of each breast, they adjust the amount they produce so that they don't continue to produce much more than he needs. As a result, he will almost fully empty each breast and will therefore automatically get both the foremilk and the hindmilk.

One breast or two?
Mothers used to use both breasts at every feed, roughly dividing the

feeding time into two equal halves between the breasts. However, as stated in the previous pages, the current thinking on foremilk and hindmilk has resulted in many mothers being told (wrongly) that they must only use one breast at each feed (to be sure that the baby gets to the hindmilk), leaving the other breast untouched for the next feed.

Although using only one breast per feed works well for mothers who are producing masses of milk, most women find that a single breast does not provide enough milk for their baby. I am frequently consulted by mothers who are worried that they don't have enough milk and, more often than not, I find that they are using only one breast per feed. These mothers don't realise that they can and should start using the second breast if there is not enough milk for their baby in the first breast. So, my advice to any mother who thinks she is short of milk is this – before resorting to giving formula, you should try offering your baby the second breast. You will usually find that this will make a big difference both to his sleeping and weight gain and you may discover that you do in fact have plenty of milk for your baby.

This is what you should do:

- Allow your baby to feed on the first breast for as long as he is sucking properly (see page 33).
- Take him off the breast and wind him.
- If he is showing all the signs of being fully fed, you can put him down to sleep.
- If, however, he is looking even remotely awake and hungry, you should offer him the second breast.
- If your baby only needs a few minutes on the second breast, that's fine, but it is equally all right to let him spend as long on the second breast as he did on the first.
- When he no longer wants to feed on the second breast, you can settle him down to sleep.

If your baby settles well and doesn't need feeding again for a reasonable amount of time (roughly three to four hours) you will know that all is well. If he doesn't do this, you will need to encourage him to feed a bit longer on one or both of your breasts – when he has had enough milk, he should be contented.

Ideally you should alternate the breast you start on so that each breast gets plenty of stimulation to encourage them to maintain a good milk supply. Keeping notes or pinning a small safety pin to your bra will remind you which breast to start with at the next feed.

Note: Many mothers only need to use one breast per feed initially, but then find that this stops being enough and they start needing to use both. So do be aware that things can change and you may need to make regular adjustments to the way you feed.

Afterpains when feeding

Afterpains are cramp-like abdominal pains which affect some mothers as they breast-feed. They can vary from being quite mild (like period pains) to being really quite strong (like labour contractions), causing considerable discomfort. These pains are caused by your uterus contracting as you feed, which means that your breast-feeding is actually helping to speed up the return of the uterus to its normal size. As this is one of the benefits of breast-feeding you should try to view these pains with a positive attitude. Afterpains normally only occur in the first few days after the birth but if you find they are causing you too much discomfort, it is fine to take a mild painkiller, such as paracetamol.

Note: First-time mothers rarely experience strong afterpains, but these frequently occur when feeding subsequent babies. They also tend to become stronger and more noticeable with every baby you have.

3 How to do a breast-feed

Some mothers find it very easy to bring their baby to the breast, while others have to learn how to do it. A baby put to the breast correctly will normally (but by no means always) know instinctively how to latch on and suck. But a baby put to the breast incorrectly is unlikely to know how to adjust the way he sucks (in order for him to get the milk quickly and easily) and may even find it quite hard to latch on at all. The main reason for this is that human breasts, unlike animal teats, tend to come in all shapes and sizes, with some shapes being much harder for a baby to latch on to. For a breast to release milk efficiently, the baby has to be latched on correctly.

Anyone who has seen an animal (such as a cow or a goat) being milked by hand will know that there is a right and a wrong way to do it. It's no good just grabbing the animal's udder and squeezing hard because, if you were to do this, not only would no milk come out but the animal would find it painful and try to move away. It is only by holding the udder in the right place and squeezing with a slow rhythmic action that any milk will come out at all and, the better the technique, the better the milk will flow.

In the same way, it's no good just sticking a baby on the breast and assuming that he will feed perfectly. Breasts, like udders, have to be milked properly in order for the milk to flow well. For this reason I think that by far the most important factor when it comes to breast-feeding is *how* you latch your baby on the breast. When a baby is latched on perfectly, he can feed calmly and easily, the mother should experience no pain or discomfort and the feeds will normally last less than one hour. It is only when the baby is incorrectly positioned that problems start to occur. So, if you can get your feeding right from the very first day, you will get off to a good start and will be unlikely to suffer from any of the problems that many mothers associate with breast-feeding.

Unfortunately, one of the biggest problems for a new mother is being able to tell the difference between a baby that is correctly positioned at the breast and one that is incorrectly positioned. This is why I am devoting an entire chapter to this subject. The main thing to bear in mind is that breast-feeding should not hurt so if it is hurting, you are almost certainly doing it incorrectly!

The ideal breast-feeding position

The following simple guidelines should ensure the best possible feed for your baby:

- The baby should be lying on his side with his body well supported (preferably by a pillow).
- His mouth should be level with the nipple.
- The nipple should be going straight into his mouth, i.e. without being pulled out of shape.
- The whole nipple and most of the areola should be in his mouth to enable his jaws to reach the reservoir of milk that is behind the nipple.
- He should be held so close that his nose touches the breast as he feeds.
- His lips should be curled back so that he is sucking on the breast rather than chewing on the nipple.
- His tongue should be positioned under the nipple, not up on the roof of his mouth.

How your baby gets the milk

Your baby needs to be latched on properly not only to enable him to get a good flow of milk but also to prevent you from getting sore nipples. Latching him on correctly will be less important if you have a fast let-down reflex, as your milk will tend to flow out of its own accord. But it will be absolutely vital if you have a slow let-down, as your milk will come out even more slowly (and in some cases it won't come out at all) if he is not sucking well and efficiently.

For your baby to get to the milk, he needs to be latched on in a way that enables his jaws to reach the collecting area behind the nipple where the milk is stored. To do this he needs to have the whole of the nipple and most of the areola in his mouth. He also needs to be very close to your breast so that he is not pulling your nipple as he sucks. If he doesn't take enough nipple in his mouth he may end up chewing on the end of it, which will almost certainly make you sore and will also frustrate him because he won't be getting much milk.

He also needs to get on at the correct angle so that your nipple is going straight into his mouth and is not being bent or pulled crookedly as he sucks. If he comes on at even slightly the wrong angle, the tiny milk ducts inside the nipple can kink and stop the milk flowing properly, in the same way that kinking a hosepipe will slow the flow of water. The more the nipple is bent out of shape, the slower the milk will flow, the longer the feeds will take and the more sore you will get. If a baby is on very crookedly the milk may not come out at all, with the result that he will want to feed for hours on end and yet will seem just as hungry at the end of the feed as he was at the start.

Doing a breast-feed

Feeding a baby is pretty much like everything else in life – if we do it correctly, it tends to work well and if we do it incorrectly, it doesn't. For this reason, you will find it much easier to feed and settle your baby if you feed in an orderly way rather than just bunging him on the breast at totally random times throughout the day and night. Although it would seem reasonable to assume that a baby will wake to feed whenever he's hungry and will stop feeding when he's had enough, an experienced mother will tell you that it's not like this at all! This is because:

- A baby wakes for all sorts of reasons other than hunger and yet will nearly always feed if you offer him the breast.
- A baby will often fall sound asleep during a feed long before he has had enough milk.
- You may spend ages winding your baby and fail to bring up any wind, and then find that he cries with wind as soon as you try to settle him.

To avoid all this confusion, I recommend that you go through a little checklist at every feed and try to do most feeds in this order:

1. Change your baby's nappy.
2. Sit comfortably.
3. Put your baby in a comfortable position.
4. Latch him on carefully.
5. Keep feeding him until he won't feed any more – do not stop the second he dozes off.

When you have finished feeding your baby, you should:

● wind him, even if he is asleep
● swaddle him firmly and then settle him down to sleep.

Having done the feed in this order your baby should have had all his needs met and is therefore less likely to start crying as soon as you lie him down, leaving you in a panic as to whether he needs more food, more winding, etc. The guidelines given above will not lead to perfect feeds and perfect babies, but it should help a lot.

Changing the nappy
A baby's nappy needs to be changed frequently, both to keep him comfortable and to prevent him getting nappy rash. As a general rule, you should change his nappy at every feed and also in between feeds if a dirty nappy wakes him up – you don't need to change it if he stays asleep. Mothers who keep their baby in a cot beside their bed will often not bother to do a nappy change in the middle of the night because it involves getting out of bed. This is fine as long as your baby is comfortable and you are using a good barrier cream, e.g. zinc and castor oil. But if he starts getting sore and developing a nappy rash, you will need to change his nappy more often, including at all the night feeds.

If at all possible, try to do the nappy change at the start of a feed because by the end, he is likely to be nice and sleepy and the last thing you will want to do is to wake him up by changing his nappy – you will usually find that he won't go back to sleep very easily and you may then need to feed him a little bit longer just to settle him again.

However, it is not worth changing the nappy at the start of each feed if:

● Your baby regularly falls sound asleep at the breast before he has taken a full feed – you'll usually find that changing his nappy at this point will wake him far more successfully to allow you to continue his feed than continually tweaking his fingers and toes.

● Your baby almost invariably does a dirty nappy during feeds. It's a waste of time and nappies always to do two nappy changes at each feed.

Sitting comfortably

As a breast-feed can last anything from 10 minutes to an hour it is important to find somewhere you can sit comfortably for the duration of the feed. However, this does not mean that you have to tuck yourself away in a remote part of the house. I say this because I regularly visit mothers who have decided that they can only feed in one room in the house, usually because this is where their feeding chair is, so they are often doing feeds sitting alone without anyone to keep them company. This is not a good idea because it can become very lonely and demoralising to sit on your own, desperately trying to speed up the feed so you can join the rest of the household.

In fact, a special feeding/nursing chair is not essential as you may find that you can be perfectly comfortable sitting in bed or on any suitable armchair or sofa, with your back well supported by cushions. However, if you cannot achieve a good level of comfort and support with your existing furniture, it is certainly worth buying a feeding chair, as they are specially designed to help to prevent backache, which is an extremely common problem for breast-feeding mothers.

Putting your baby in a comfortable position

Make your baby comfortable by lying him in such a way that he can feed easily from the breast without having to crane his neck and strain to reach your nipple. The best way to achieve this is to use several pillows to bring him to the level of your breasts and then to lie him on the top one so that his body is totally supported by it. This will tend to be much more comfortable for him than the more traditional method of cradling him on an arm. It will also make it much easier for him to latch on correctly. Although some mothers can feed very successfully by cradling their babies on their arms, I find that most of the mothers I see doing this are not getting it right and subsequently find it much easier to feed using pillows. This is especially the case if they have particularly large breasts or rather flat nipples, either of which can make latching on much more difficult.

How to use pillows

Once you are sitting comfortably you will need to fill the gap between your lap and your breasts with pillows. The number of pillows you use will depend upon how big that gap is. Some mothers find they only need one pillow (once their breast is released from a good supporting bra!) while others will need two or three. Be sure to arrange the pillows carefully so that they support your baby fully throughout the feed and, if necessary, place a pillow to the side of your body to provide extra support for the top pillow to rest on. You will probably need this extra pillow when feeding in bed or on a sofa when you are feeding on the breast away from the armrest.

● Tuck the top pillow as close into your body as possible by lifting your breast with one hand and using the other hand to pull the pillow right in against your ribcage. See below.

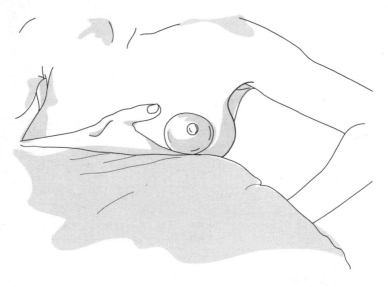

Lifting the breast

● Rest your breast back down on to the pillow so that your nipple is as far into the centre of the pillow as possible. The reason for doing this is to allow your baby to lie on the centre bit of the pillow, which is firm and will support him well, rather than having him falling off the edge. See opposite.

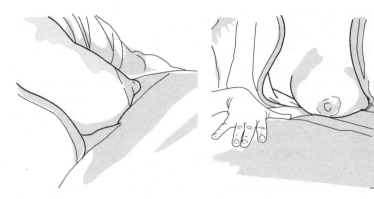

*Placing the breast on a pillow
(side view)*

*Placing the breast on a pillow
(front view)*

● Lie your baby on his side with his mouth an inch away from your
nipple, then let go of him. If he remains in exactly the same
position, with his mouth still next to your nipple you will know
you've got your pillows right. See below.

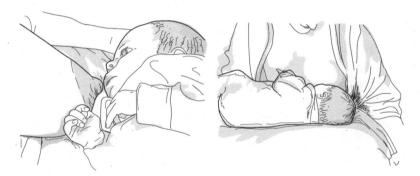

*Baby lying with mouth directly in
front of nipple*

*Lying your baby on his side (front
view)*

Latching your baby on

Most babies are born with a very strong sucking reflex and will
automatically suck on anything that is put near their mouth. However,
I do fairly regularly come across a baby who doesn't seem to have
this natural instinct and needs a bit more help. If a baby like this is
presented with breasts that are not an ideal shape it is even harder
for him to latch on naturally and the mother will need to be quite skilful
to help him to get on the breast (see Baby can't latch on, page 102).

The most important thing to keep in mind is that you should bring the baby to the breast, not the breast to the baby. I often see a mother perched on the edge of a chair bending over her baby, desperately trying to heave a large breast into his mouth, which is at least six inches away from where her breast belongs! If she does manage to get him latched on in this way, she will usually spend the rest of the feed hunched over him and will often develop backache, neck ache and sore nipples as a result of this uncomfortable feeding position.

So, when it comes to latching, I would advise the following:

- Sit comfortably and arrange your pillows to the correct height.
- Lie your baby on the top pillow, not on your arm.
- Lie him on his side, with his tummy close to your body and his mouth directly in front of your nipple (see page 29).
- Hold him firmly (but not roughly) so that you have good control of his head.
- If your baby is crying (and his mouth is therefore wide open!) move him swiftly towards your breast so that you can get as much of your nipple in his mouth as possible *before* he closes it and starts sucking.
- If his mouth is shut, try brushing your nipple against his lips – this should cause him to open his mouth by stimulating the 'rooting reflex'.
- Once he has successfully latched on, hold him close as he feeds (his nose should touch your breast) so that he is not pulling your nipple towards his mouth. (see below).

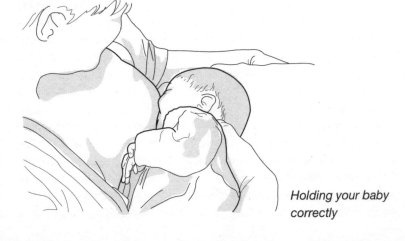

Holding your baby correctly

When your baby first latches on, you may get a bit of a shock as the first few sucks will feel surprisingly strong, but after a while he should settle down into slow, rhythmic sucking that doesn't hurt at all. If it does hurt or if you feel any strong pulling, you are not doing it right and you must correct the problem before continuing to feed.

How will I know if my baby is latched on properly?
Once your baby has done a few sucks you should check to see whether he has latched on properly before you carry on feeding; all of your nipple and most of the areola should have disappeared into his mouth. You should not feel any pulling as your baby sucks (this would indicate that he is either not close enough to the breast or that he is on crookedly) and it certainly should not hurt. Don't be fooled into thinking that the harder you feel your baby sucking, the better he is sucking, because when a baby is latched on properly you should hardly be able to feel him suck at all. A mother will often proudly tell me that she has sore nipples because her baby has such a good, strong suck – she is then rather disappointed when I explain that strong sucking is more an indication of incorrect positioning than a sign that her baby is very clever!

The four main points to look out for are:

1. *Has your baby got enough nipple and areola in his mouth?*
The amount of areola that your baby will be able to get in his mouth will depend upon how large your nipples are. If you have tiny nipples, he should latch on, taking the entire nipple and all the areola into his mouth so that once he starts sucking no areola is visible. If, on the other hand, you have extremely large nipples, he should still take the whole nipple into his mouth but probably won't manage to take all the areola as well – as he sucks you may see some areola that is not covered by his lips. Irrespective of how much nipple and areola is in your baby's mouth, he should have his mouth wide open and his lips curled back – see Correctly latched on, page 32.

If your baby latches on without taking enough nipple in his mouth (see Incorrectly latched on, page 32) you will need to take him off and start again because once his jaw is clamped shut you cannot shovel more soft nipple into his mouth! Never pull your baby off without first breaking the suction – to do this will almost certainly result in sore nipples. Instead, take him off by putting one of your

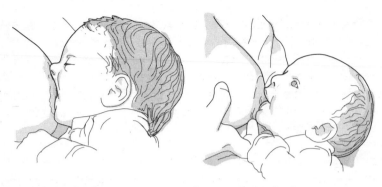

Correctly latched on   *Incorrectly latched on*

fingers into his mouth and sliding it between his gums so that he has fully released your nipple before you pull him away from your breast. Do not lick your finger before you put it in his mouth. Not only is this unnecessary but your saliva might contain bacteria that is harmful to a small baby. Try putting him on again but if he keeps latching on incorrectly you may need to help him by shaping your nipple. (See Baby can't latch on, page 102.)

2. *Are you holding your baby close enough?*
One of the most common mistakes mothers make is to have their baby too far away from the breast (for fear of blocking his nose), which results in a lot of pulling of the nipple and a poor milk flow. As you feed you should have your baby's face so close to your breast that he can suck without having to pull your nipple towards his mouth – if your nipple is being pulled towards his mouth, his gums will not be reaching the milk reservoir behind the nipple. To achieve this closeness, you may need to have your baby's nose almost buried in your breast. Don't worry about his being unable to breathe if you hold him this close – babies' noses are designed to allow them to feed like this. But if you were to hold him so close that he really couldn't breathe, he would soon let you know by stopping feeding and pulling away from the breast. A baby will not carry on sucking if he can't breathe through his nose.

3. *Is your baby on at the correct angle?*
If your baby is on at slightly the wrong angle, each suck will hurt, you will notice a lot of puckering of your breast around the nipple and it will feel as if your breast is being pulled towards your baby's mouth.

If this happens, look at your breast to see where the pulling is coming from, then gently move him towards the direction of the pull while he continues to suck. As soon as you get your baby into the correct feeding position you should feel the pulling stop. Once you are satisfied that your baby is on properly, and nothing is hurting, relax your shoulders and let him carry on feeding. (See also Different feeding positions, page 41.)

4. *Is he sucking correctly?*
When a baby latches on correctly he will normally suck in the same sort of way that he would on a bottle. In other words, he will often start with some fairly short quick sucks and then, once the milk starts to flow, his sucks will become slower, deeper and more rhythmic in action. When he does this, you should notice that his whole jaw is moving and this movement should extend right up the jaw line as far as his ears. You would also expect him to keep feeding fairly continuously for a good 10 minutes or so without the need for you to stroke his cheek or tickle his feet to keep him going. Signs of poor sucking are:

● Pursed lips and hollowed cheeks.
● Small, infrequent and shallow sucks.
● Falling asleep at the breast (because he is not being rewarded with a good milk flow).

How will I know when my baby has had enough milk?
Life would be so much simpler if breasts worked like a gasometer and visibly deflated with each ounce of milk that the baby extracts! But unfortunately they don't work like this, so it's impossible to know exactly how much milk a baby has had at any point during a feed. In fact, the best way to judge whether he is getting enough milk is to see how long he lasts between one feed and the next – the longer he lasts, the more milk he is likely to have had. You can also weigh him regularly to see whether he is putting on weight. Both these methods mean that you will only know whether he has had enough milk in retrospect, i.e. when he wakes for the next feed or when you weigh him. It's therefore a question of exercising your judgement, rather than having anything more scientific to go by.

There are, however, several signs to look out for before, during and after a feed that will give you some clues. These are:

- If you feel your breast before you start feeding it will normally feel firm and quite full.
- As the feed progresses, your breast will become softer and feel less full.
- When the breast is nearly (or completely) empty, it will feel very soft.
- At the start of a feed when your baby is hungry, you would expect him to suck strongly and almost continuously with very few pauses.
- As his tummy fills up with milk, his sucking will tend to slow and he will start pausing a lot more.
- When you reach the point at which your baby is doing almost as much pausing as sucking, you can assume that he has emptied your breast and/or had enough milk.

Although you still won't know exactly how much milk he has had, the above signs would indicate that your baby has done a pretty good job of emptying the first breast and it's time to wind him and then offer him the second breast. He *may* now have had enough milk and be ready to go to sleep, but you should still try and wake him to see whether he will feed for a bit longer. If he does latch onto the second breast and suck eagerly and regularly (i.e. he is not just 'comfort-sucking'), you should carry on feeding him until his sucking slows and he is once again doing more pausing than sucking. At this point, you can still try to stimulate him to feed more continuously but if he doesn't start sucking strongly again he may finally have had enough milk. Even if he is sound asleep, don't make the mistake of trying to settle him without winding him first, because this will almost invariably result in his waking shortly after you have put him down to sleep.

If your baby remains sleepy after burping, you can settle him down and keep your fingers crossed that you have not misread the signals and that he has indeed had enough milk. But if the winding process wakes him up again, try putting him back to the breast to see if he wants more food. When you reach the stage where he either doesn't want to feed at all or is only feeding for a minute or two when you put him back to the breast, you can try to settle him down to sleep. You won't know for sure that he has had enough milk, but there comes a point when it is not worth carrying on feeding if he is spending more time dozing than sucking.

Time how long the feed lasted and see how long your baby sleeps until the next feed. If he stays asleep for a reasonable amount of time (e.g. three to four hours) you will know that you got it right. If, however, he wakes with hunger after only about two hours, you should try to keep him feeding for a bit longer at the next feed. You can do this by feeding him in a cooler room, having him less warmly clothed or by doing your nappy change halfway through the feed rather than at the start of the feed.

You can expect it to take you several days (at least) before you begin to recognise when your baby has had enough milk and for you to know approximately how long it takes *your* baby to empty *your* breasts.

You will know your baby is getting enough milk if:

- He settles well after feeds.
- He sleeps reasonably well in between feeds.
- He is putting on the right amount of weight.

Winding

There is a myth that breast-fed babies don't need winding, but I'm afraid that this is certainly not true – a breast-fed baby will often need just as much winding as a bottle-fed baby, especially if he is badly attached to the breast. However, a *small* proportion of babies do not suffer from wind at all and, if your baby falls into this category, you will not need to wind him as described below.

When a baby feeds, he will usually swallow some air, which then starts accumulating in his tummy as wind. The more air he takes in, the more uncomfortable he will feel and the more frequently he will need winding.

Although the amount of wind a baby suffers from rarely seems to bear any relation to whether he is breast-fed or bottle-fed, some babies do seem to suffer more from wind than others, and some are definitely much harder to wind than others. You should always wind a baby at the end of a feed and also at any point during a feed when he seems uncomfortable. You need to do this for the following reasons:

- A baby with too much wind in his tummy can become too uncomfortable to carry on feeding.
- Air in his tummy can sometimes make him feel full and may stop him feeding before he has had enough milk.

- Winding a baby firmly will usually wake him up if he has fallen asleep before he has had enough milk – a baby will often doze off when his tummy is only half-full.
- If your baby *does* wake up when you wind him, you will need put him back to the breast to see whether he wants to feed for a bit longer.
- Winding a baby at the end of each feed is essential because a baby will rarely settle for long if he still has wind in his tummy. Even a baby who appears to be sound asleep will tend to wake and start crying within minutes if you lie him down without first winding him.

How to wind your baby

The air bubbles trapped in a baby's tummy will only be able to come up easily when his back is straight, thus allowing the wind a free passage up. Most mothers are advised to sit their babies on their lap when winding (see below). This may well work for you, but you may find that your baby ends up in a crumpled heap with his back bent, in which case it will take much longer to wind him than if his back is nice and straight.

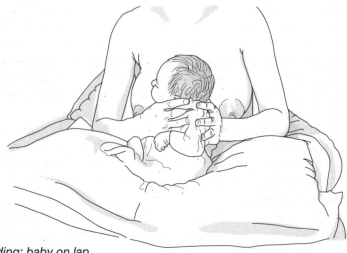

Winding: baby on lap

I find that the best way to wind a baby is to hold his body firmly against my chest with one hand, while using the other hand to push gently into the small of his back to make sure it is completely straight (see opposite).

Winding: holding baby against chest

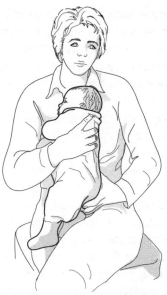

Another easy way is to lie him over your shoulder and pat or rub his back. This works well as it does ensure that his back is straight, but the disadvantage of this method is that you may end up with a lot of extra washing if your baby sicks up some milk onto your clothes. It is very common and normal for a baby to bring up a small amount of milk when he burps – this is called possetting. You will, however, usually find that he will tend to bring up more milk if you wind him when applying pressure on his tummy than he would if you winded him by holding him against your chest.

You will find that it will take quite a few feeds before you get to know when to stop and wind your baby. This can vary enormously from baby to baby – some will happily go an entire feed without needing winding, while others may need winding at regular intervals throughout the feed.

The amount of time that you need to spend winding your baby will depend entirely on how easy he is to wind. Normally, a baby will burp within a minute or two of winding, but if this doesn't happen, you will need to wind him for longer. However, it doesn't matter if he doesn't bring up wind when he is winded during the middle of a feed. If he starts crying before he has done a burp and seems to want to get on with feeding, you can put him back to the breast and finish winding him at the end of the feed.

As a general rule, I suggest that at the end of each feed you spend a maximum of 10 minutes winding your baby – if he hasn't brought up wind within this time it's usually not worth carrying on. However, if you do end up settling him without bringing up any wind, you may well find that he starts crying soon after you lie him down. If this happens, wind will be the most likely cause of his crying, so you should pick him up and have another go.

How will I know whether I have got all the wind up?
The short answer is – you won't! It is really a question of trial and error to begin with because you cannot assume that, once a baby has done one burp, there are no more to come. However, as you get to know your baby, you will discover for yourself whether he never needs winding, whether he is fully winded after only one burp or whether it takes several burps before all his wind is up.

Useful tip: When a baby has wind, his back will usually curve outwards and his spine will resist your efforts to straighten it. When a baby has little or no wind, his spine will feel very flexible and he won't resist when you press the small of his back.

Hiccups
It is very common for a baby to have hiccups. Most babies are completely untroubled by them and will happily carry on with whatever they are doing, e.g. feeding, sleeping, etc. But if you find that your baby *is* unsettled with hiccups, you could try offering him some cool boiled water (either from a bottle or from a spoon) to see if this helps.

Swaddling
A baby will normally sleep longer and better if he is firmly wrapped in a nice warm swaddling sheet than he will if he is not swaddled. Unfortunately, many mothers are now advised not to swaddle their babies (for fear of overheating them) and these mothers will usually find that their babies tend to sleep less soundly than their swaddled counterparts. This is because a baby put down to sleep without a swaddling sheet will often be woken in between feeds by involuntary jerks (which are both common and normal) of their arms or legs.

It is a shame not to swaddle your baby because, having spent the last few months of the pregnancy being squashed up in your womb, he will feel cosy and protected if he can spend a few more weeks feeling equally secure. You will also find it much easier to keep him warm in winter if you wrap him up cosily in a swaddling sheet, rather than just piling blankets on top of him.

Of course when it comes to the question of overheating your baby you must use your common sense. If you swaddled him on a hot summer's day, for example, you would need to adjust his clothing (on a really hot day, possibly just a nappy would do) and you would swaddle him using a cotton sheet rather than a blanket or shawl. In a real heatwave, you should not swaddle your baby.

The same criteria would apply in the winter. You should not have the central heating on full blast and your baby dressed in many layers of vests, babygros, etc., if you are also swaddling him. The big advantage of swaddling in the winter (apart from your baby sleeping better) is that your heating bills will be reduced and you won't need to spend ages dressing him in layers of clothing.

Your midwife at the hospital will be able to show you how to swaddle your baby – see page 40. I expect your mother will also know how to swaddle a baby as she probably swaddled you when you were a baby. You can carry on swaddling your baby for as long as it suits him, which will usually be for at least six weeks. When he becomes agitated and fights against being so tightly wrapped you will know the time has come to stop.

To swaddle your baby effectively, you will need a swaddling sheet (obtainable from most shops) or thin blanket or shawl that is big enough to wrap tightly round his body without it all coming undone as soon as he wriggles.

How to swaddle your baby
1. Take your swaddling sheet and fold one corner down.
2. Lie the baby on the cloth so that his neck is on the crease – see page 40 (a).
3. Bring up the corner A of the cloth and wrap it over and under your baby – see page 40 (b).
4. Bring up corner B from the bottom as shown – see page 40 (c).
5. Bring corner C over and tuck it under his body – see page 40 (d).

Once your baby is firmly swaddled, settle him down to sleep either on his side or on his back but never lying on his tummy – research has shown that this might be a contributory factor to cot death. If you lie him on his side, you can place a small rolled-up towel on either side of his body to stop him rolling over.

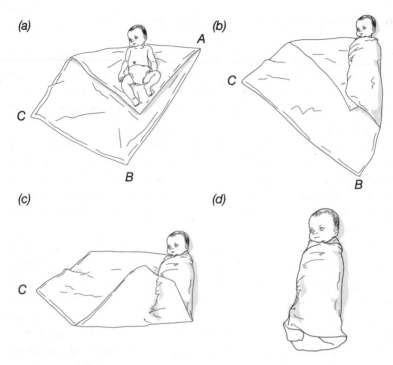

Note: If your baby clearly hates having his arms confined or has reached the stage where he wants to suck his thumb, it is still worth swaddling him but you can wrap him up leaving his arms free.

Settling your baby after feeds

Some babies settle quickly and easily after feeds, some take a long time to fall asleep and some find it almost impossible to go to sleep without some help. You won't know which category your baby comes into until you start trying to put him down to sleep. There are several steps you should take before attempting to settle your baby. Above all, you need to be clear in your own mind that sleep is the one and only thing he needs so that you can concentrate on getting him to sleep without worrying about whether he needs more winding or food, etc.

With this in mind you should:

● Keep on feeding your baby for as long as he is prepared to feed properly, i.e. he should not just be sucking for pleasure.
● Change his nappy if necessary.
● Wind him for as long as is necessary bring up a burp, or for up to 10 minutes.

● Swaddle your baby so that he feels secure.

Once you have been through this checklist you should place him in his Moses basket, crib or pram to see whether he goes straight to sleep. If he does, that's all you have to do. If he lies awake but is not crying, you can leave him either until he goes to sleep or until he starts crying.

If your baby starts crying *gently*, your first course of action is to do nothing! Leave him for up to 10 minutes to see whether he goes to sleep of his own accord – it's not cruel to do this as many babies will only fall asleep if they are left to cry. If you keep picking up a crying baby you may end up making him thoroughly overtired and even more incapable of going to sleep.

If your baby goes to sleep within the 10 minutes you will have learnt a valuable lesson! If, however, he is still crying but the crying remains at the same level or starts diminishing, you can leave him for a little bit longer to see if he falls asleep. At this point, you could try offering him a dummy and it might help if you rock his crib and/or gently pat his back. If his crying escalates, or if he is still crying after 10 minutes or so, you will need to pick him up to wind him again and calm him down.

Once you have done this, try to settle him down again, but if absolutely nothing (i.e. winding, rocking or dummy) settles him, you will need to go back to square one to see whether he needs more milk. If he does, this will probably explain why he wouldn't go to sleep, and you should find that he settles once you have fed him a bit more. However, if he still won't settle, he may have a problem that needs attending to (e.g. colic, see page 144).

Note: If you establish that leaving your baby to cry himself to sleep never works (and merely serves to get him thoroughly upset each time you try), you should not continue to put either him or yourself through the distress of continuing with this method. I would also emphasise that you should only leave your baby to cry if you are fairly confident that you have met all his needs and that he is ready to go to sleep.

Different feeding positions

Although I suggest that all new mothers should at least start off by using the feeding position that I recommend (see The ideal breast-feeding position, page 24), there are several other ways of feeding your baby that can work perfectly well, provided they are done correctly. My main objection to these other methods is that they tend to make a mother much more likely to latch her baby on incorrectly. Nonetheless, I fully accept that a woman with no breast-feeding problems can happily use some or all of the methods that are described below.

Cradling in your arm

This is the method most commonly used by breast-feeding mothers and, when done correctly, it is comfortable for both mother and baby. The important thing to realise when using this method is that your baby's head should lie halfway down your arm (see below) and should not be cradled in the crook of your arm – this will tilt his head the wrong way and make it difficult for him to latch on easily. Putting a pillow or small cushion under your arm while you feed will help to support the weight of your baby and will take some of the strain off your arm.

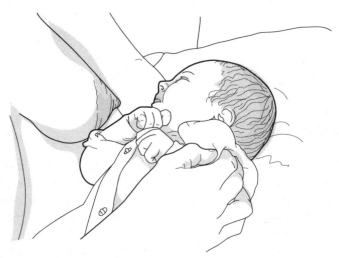

Cradling him halfway down your arm

As with all methods of feeding, you should sit in a position that is comfortable for you, so that you do not develop backache or a stiff neck as the feed progresses. Any chair, sofa or bed that provides good support for your back should be fine, and a special feeding/nursing chair is ideal, though not essential.

The football hold

This is the method a mother with twins will use to breast-feed her babies simultaneously and is, in my opinion, virtually the only time the football hold should be used. This is because this method of feeding involves tucking your baby under your arm (see below) and it is very hard to do this without him being pushed out of position when his feet touch the surface you are leaning against, e.g. the back of the chair. The football hold only works well if you position yourself well forward (using pillows to support your back) so that there is enough room for your baby's feet to extend beyond your back.

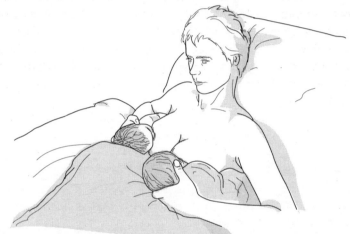

The football hold

Many mothers are advised to try using the football hold if they are suffering from problems such as sore nipples or blocked milk ducts, on the basis that changing the feeding position will often resolve the problem. It's certainly true that changing the angle at which you feed your baby will help these conditions, but only if the new approach helps you to latch your baby on 100 per cent correctly. What most mothers find is that, while the football hold initially appears to help make feeds less painful, after a few feeds they realise that all they have done is transfer the problem to a different part of the breast. For this reason, a mother suffering from sore nipples or blocked milk ducts will usually find that it is better to try altering the feeding position while her baby is lying on a pillow in front of her (as described in previous chapters) rather than changing to the football hold and just hoping that it will be the miracle answer.

However, every now and then I will come across a baby who, for some obscure reason, feeds perfectly well on one breast but refuses point-blank to feed on the other. As far as I can judge, the baby seems to have developed a phobia for that particular breast, but can be fooled into feeding on it if you use the football hold. I usually find that such a baby will happily revert to feeding normally on that breast after only five minutes or so of using this hold. If you use the football hold for a baby like this, it is essential to put him on the breast very quickly, before he realises what is going on! It is therefore important to get yourself ready in advance by arranging cushions behind your back, enabling you to sit well forward in the chair.

Note: If your baby continues to reject a particular breast whenever you try to feed him without using the football hold, you could consider consulting a cranial osteopath (see page 178) to see whether there is a physical reason why he cannot feed on that side.

Lying down

Mothers often ask me whether it is all right to feed their baby lying down on their side in bed. As a general rule it is not something that I recommend as, like the football hold, it can be quite hard to latch a baby on correctly and easily in this position. However, some breasts are better suited than others to feeding like this (size and shape make a big difference) so I am certainly not against feeding when lying on your side, provided you can do it without causing any trauma to your nipples and provided you stay awake. If however, you develop sore nipples or find that the feed takes much longer (which would indicate that the baby is not latched on correctly) whenever you do it lying down, you should try altering positions or abandon this way of feeding altogether.

You should also consider the following:

● Research by the Foundation for the Study of Infant Deaths has shown that babies taken into the parental bed for any reason *are* at a greater risk of cot death (see page 62).
● A mother will often choose to feed her baby while lying down so that she can snatch 40 winks during the feed – and she will usually find that her baby dozes off to sleep as well. This can seem like a real bonus in the middle of the night but it is actually for this latter reason (i.e. the baby falling asleep) that I am most against feeding like this. If your baby regularly falls asleep before

he has taken an adequate feed, your breasts will be under-stimulated (and will start producing less milk) and your baby will find it hard to catch up on his milk intake later on in the day. It can also result in a baby becoming used to falling asleep within the warm confines of his mother's body, and then not being at all keen to be put to sleep elsewhere, e.g. in a Moses basket. So, what at the time may seem like a good solution to help a desperately tired mother with an unsettled baby can actually result in longer-term problems that can become equally demoralising to deal with at a later date.

- A mother who has had her baby delivered by Caesarean section may think that it will be less painful to feed him lying on her side rather than sitting up. In fact, if you sit comfortably with your baby lying on a pillow (see page 27) this will stop any pressure being put on your scar and you should find this easier and less painful than any other way of feeding.

If, despite all of the above, you do decide to try feeding your baby lying on your side, it is really a question of trial and error, experimenting with different positions to find out which is the most comfortable for you and your baby. See below for ideas.

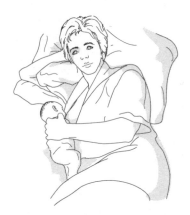

Breast-feeding on your side using the lower breast

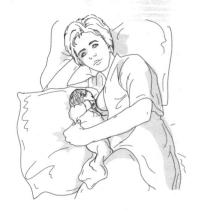

Breast-feeding on your side using a pillow to bring the baby to the level of the upper breast

4 The first few days

This chapter describes in detail what you can expect to happen on the breast-feeding front during the first few days. If breast-feeding goes well right from the word go, the mother is not only filled with confidence but is also unlikely to find that she subsequently develops problems. But if a mother does have problems in the first few days she will usually find it fairly traumatic and may well feel that, if this is what breast-feeding is all about, she would rather bottle-feed. With this in mind, I will try to cover in this chapter all the different problems that a mother might encounter and explain various ways to avoid the problem occurring in the first place.

When your baby is born

Your baby's first feed will usually be on the labour ward, with the midwife who delivered you being there to help you and show you how it's done. Ideally, you would feed your baby within an hour of his birth, but if he doesn't want to feed or you are too tired after a long labour, it is perfectly all right to wait until you get down to the post-natal ward. Your midwife will be able to advise you on this.

The first 24 hours

Some babies are very hungry and wakeful after the birth and start feeding immediately, while others are very sleepy and may not want to feed much to begin with. If your baby falls into the first category, you can ignore the rest of this section and turn straight to Before your milk comes in, page 55.

If your baby does not start feeding immediately and fairly regularly, you should note which of these categories he comes into:

- Your baby latches on and feeds well, but only has about three feeds in the first 24 hours. This is normal and you need not be concerned that he is feeding so infrequently. You should, however, expect him to feed at least six times a day after this initial period of calm.

- He spends the first 12 hours or so sleeping and shows no sign of either wanting or needing to feed. Your midwife is aware of this but is not concerned, as your baby is clearly healthy and will probably start feeding as and when he needs to.

- He spends the first 12 hours or so sleeping and shows no sign of wanting to feed but your midwife *is* slightly concerned. If your baby is 'jittery' (a sign that he needs food) your midwife might do a blood test to check his glucose levels. If they are low, your midwife will almost certainly suggest that you wake him and try to get him to feed on the breast. If, however, they are within the normal range, she may feel that it is all right to let him go another few hours without a feed. If in doubt, a paediatrician should be consulted.

- Your baby keeps crying and clearly wants to feed but is unable to latch onto your breast. This tends to happen to mothers who have very large breasts or large flat nipples, which make it much harder for a baby to latch on. **It is vital to differentiate between a baby who does not *need* to feed and a baby who is *trying* to feed but cannot.** Every effort should be made to get this baby onto the breast (as he clearly both wants and needs milk) and you should either enlist the help of an experienced midwife or refer to Baby can't latch on, page 102.

  If he is still unable to latch onto the breast you could try to express your colostrum by hand (see Expressing milk, page 89) and he can then be given this using a small syringe. If you are unable to express enough colostrum, your baby may need to be given some formula milk – discuss this with the midwife and/or a paediatrician.

If your baby has still not fed at all after about 12 hours (regardless of whether or not he's been trying to feed), you should start taking a more active role to get him feeding.

The main reasons for doing this are:

- Not all babies will wake regularly for feeds (especially if you had painkilling drugs towards the end of your labour, which will make your baby sleepy), so you can't always assume that a sleeping baby does not need feeding.

- In the first few days before your milk comes in, your breasts only produce small amounts of colostrum, which allows your baby to feed little and often. If he goes for too long (for example, eight hours) without food, your breasts may not be capable of suddenly supplying eight hours' worth of colostrum in one feed.

- It is important to recognise that, on a busy post-natal ward, the midwives may be unaware that your baby has made numerous failed attempts to breast-feed and it may be up to you to let them know exactly how long he has gone without any milk.

- Some babies who go for too long without food can become too weak and apathetic to suck at the breast. This can happen even when a baby is clinically well, i.e. his blood glucose levels are within the normal range. (A classic sign that your baby is becoming weak is if he cries for a feed, latches on well but then only takes a few sucks before falling asleep.)

- The longer your baby goes without a feed, the more likely he is to become dehydrated, which in turn makes him even less able to feed. He may then stop waking at all for feeds and this is often wrongly interpreted (by inexperienced midwives and new mothers) to mean that he doesn't need feeding.

If the decision is made that your baby *should* be given some milk, I don't think it matters at all how he is given it, so long as he gets the right amount (i.e. as much as he will drink) – this would normally be at least 30 ml (1 oz). Giving your baby the milk he requires should not have any adverse effect on breast-feeding, but mothers are often made to feel that they have failed if they have to give formula at this early stage – even though it is only being given on a temporary basis. For this reason, I think it is very important that you read the following section on cup-feeding.

Cup-feeding
If your baby does need to be given some milk, the midwife will probably use a small plastic cup to feed him, rather than a bottle. This is because many people think that if a breast-fed baby is given even one bottle it will impair his sucking reflex by causing 'nipple–teat confusion', which will prevent the baby from ever

feeding successfully on the breast. This is an issue that I feel very strongly about, because mothers are given such wrong and misleading advice on this subject.

I know of many a mother who has given her baby a bottle of formula milk on the advice of a paediatrician or midwife and has then been reduced to tears by another midwife or breast-feeding counsellor berating her for doing this. The mother is told that she has now ruined all chance of her baby being able to breast-feed and is left to feel a complete failure on all counts. I cannot understand why this 'nipple–teat' theory is still being touted around, when several studies have shown that breast-fed babies *can* be given a bottle without it having an adverse effect on breast-feeding. The Royal College of Midwives actually makes a point of discussing this issue in their book on breast-feeding (which is written for midwives and other health professionals) and yet many midwives still continue to tell mothers that they must *never* give a bottle.

The upshot of all this conflicting advice is that, while I think that giving one or two feeds with a cup is probably a good idea, if your baby continues to need extra feeding I recommend that you change to using a bottle.

My reasons for this are:

● Cup-feeding requires the skill of an experienced midwife to ensure that the milk goes down the baby's throat (rather than his clothes!) and a new mother is unlikely to be this skilled.
● It can be quite frightening for a new mother to cope with cup-feeding (especially in the middle of the night), whereas bottle-feeding is easy and most mothers will feel much more confident doing this.
● It is hard to see exactly how much milk your baby is getting when you are cup-feeding, so he may end up getting less milk than he needs.
● There is no evidence to suggest that giving a few bottle feeds will confuse a breast-fed baby.
● If the reason the baby is being given a bottle is because he can't or won't breast-feed, it seems a bit illogical to blame the bottle if the baby then continues not to suck at the breast.
● I have very rarely found that a baby who has been given a bottle will subsequently refuse to suck on the breast provided he is

given the help he needs (i.e. by making the breast a better shape for him, see page 102). I also take the view that any sucking is better than no sucking at all.

In most cases, one or two cup-feeds or bottle-feeds will usually be enough to raise a baby's energy levels and help him to make a successful attempt at getting on the breast later on in the day. If this happens you should, of course, stop bottle-feeding him and settle into a normal breast-feeding pattern.

You should however be concerned that your baby is not feeding well and is becoming dehydrated if:

- He is not settling well after feeds and is constantly crying.
- He is sleepy and is not waking for feeds on a regular basis (every three to four hours).
- He is not passing enough urine; he should be wetting his nappy at least once every four hours – putting a tissue in his nappy will help you to see whether he is doing this.
- He takes less than 30 ml (1 oz) of milk if you offer him a bottle.

If any of the above happens, you should contact your district midwife or ring your local hospital for advice. If your baby has become severely dehydrated, he may need to be admitted to hospital to be given some fluids either by tube or by intravenous infusion. Although this will be very upsetting and traumatic for you, do be reassured that you will both quickly recover and you should still be able to breast-feed once your baby is back to normal.

Case History 1
Caroline Banks. Twins George and India (aged 4 days)

Caroline's twins were born two weeks early. George started feeding immediately but India was unable to latch on to the breast. The midwives were concerned because India was a small baby and her blood sugar levels were found to be low. Caroline reluctantly agreed to allow the midwives to give India cup-feeds of formula milk every three to four hours and asked her husband to ring me to ask my opinion. I was in full agreement with the midwives and was delighted to hear that India was being fed on a regular basis, albeit by cup rather than breast.

I reassured Caroline's husband that this would not affect her breast-feeding but said that I would visit her in hospital if India continued to be unable to latch on to the breast. After four days India was still being cup-fed, as a result of which the hospital was reluctant to discharge her. When I visited Caroline I asked her to show me how she was attempting to latch India on the breast and I could see immediately what the problem was. Although Caroline had small breasts, she was squeezing her breast in such a way as to make it quite difficult for India to latch on. George, being a bigger baby, was able to cope but was still not latching on very well and Caroline's nipples were becoming sore.

By shaping the breast correctly, it took all of 30 seconds to get India latched on to the breast! She needed no further cup-feeds and both she and George continued to feed so well that they were allowed home two days later.

Conclusion: *Some babies need more help than others to get on the breast. Thanks to the midwives giving regular feeds during the period when India was not latching on, India did not become tired and weak. As a result, she had no problem latching on to the breast once it was made easier for her.*

Case History 2
Helen Long and Jack (aged three days)

When Jack was born Helen found that he was unable to latch on to the breast. After two full days of failed attempts (during which time Jack was given no other milk), Helen was becoming increasingly anxious and Jack was becoming increasingly lethargic. She discussed the situation with the midwives, who decided to give Jack a cup-feed of formula milk. Then, at 2am, a keen (but misguided) midwife decided to make a concerted effort to get Jack on the breast. After one and a half hours and still no success, he was exhausted and so was Helen. He was then given another cup-feed.

Helen rang me in the morning to let me know what had gone on both during the night and over the previous two days, and I said I would come and visit her. However, I warned her that it was extremely unlikely that I would be able to get Jack to feed at the breast. He had had less than 60 ml (2 oz) of milk in three days and this, coupled with the fact that he was now having phototherapy for jaundice, meant that he was unlikely to have the energy to suck at the breast. This turned out to be the case. I was easily able to get him to latch on, but after only a couple of sucks he would fall asleep. It was very apparent that there was nothing to be gained by continuing to try to get him to feed at the breast as he was clearly far too tired. I suggested to his parents that he should have a minimum of two or three bottle-feeds to restore his energy, after which I was pretty confident that he would start breast-feeding.

Helen had very large, flat nipples, which was why Jack had found it hard to latch on. I showed her how to shape her nipple to make it easier for him, but suggested that she made no further attempt to get him on the breast for the next 12 hours or so. This was partly because I felt that he was too tired to feed properly and partly because Helen herself was tired and demoralised, and any further failed attempt at the breast might be the final straw for both of them.

Jack took 35 ml (just over 1 oz) of formula milk at the first bottle feed, after which Helen expressed milk, which was then given to him at subsequent feeds. The following morning, Jack's jaundice had dispersed; he was discharged home and by the evening he was happily feeding at the breast and needing no further bottle-feeds.

Conclusion: When a baby goes for too long without milk, he can become temporarily incapable of sucking on the breast. Giving a few feeds by bottle will usually restore his energy and is unlikely to inhibit his ability to suck at the breast.

Case History 3
Rosie Delaney and Becky (aged four days)

From the day she was born, Becky was bad at latching on to the breast. On each occasion she would latch on, take a few sucks and then fall asleep. Rosie was on a busy post-natal ward and none of the midwives realised that breast-feeding was going wrong and that Becky was getting no milk. She was discharged home on Day 3 and I went to visit her on Day 4.

By this stage, Becky was not waking for feeds and I could not get her to take even one suck at the breast. On close questioning, I established from her parents that she had had a total of 90 ml (3 oz) of formula milk since her birth four days previously. She had been given this on three separate occasions when the father had told the midwives how concerned he was that his baby did not appear to be sucking enough to get any breast milk. Becky's nappies had also been dry for at least 24 hours and she was clearly jaundiced.

All the indications were that Becky was extremely weak and dehydrated. I offered her some formula milk from a bottle but she took less than 15 ml (½ oz). On the basis of this, I recommended that her parents should take her straight to hospital. Becky was admitted immediately and was given intravenous fluids to reverse her dehydration and phototherapy to treat her jaundice. By the time she was discharged home a day or two later, Rosie was so traumatised that she decided to make no further attempt to breast-feed Becky and went on to full-time bottle-feeding.

Conclusion: *A baby needs to be fed regularly to prevent dehydration. Had Rosie realised this and alerted the midwives to the fact that Becky was not sucking properly at the breast, the crisis could have been averted and Rosie may well have succeeded in breast-feeding.*

Case History 4
Joanna Harding. Twins Lucy and Alicia (aged seven weeks)

When Joanna's twins were born, Lucy latched on immediately but, despite numerous attempts at the breast, Alicia consistently failed to latch on. She was cup-fed for several days and Joanna stayed in hospital, hoping to get breast-feeding established before she went home. Unfortunately, this did not happen so Joanna decided that, once she got home, she would continue to breast-feed Lucy but would express milk for Alicia. Joanna soon started giving Alicia all her feeds from a bottle, as cup-feeding proved to be too complicated and time-consuming.

Joanna carried on like this for seven weeks, at which point her GP suggested that she consult me. As soon as I showed Joanna how to shape her breast, Alicia latched on and sucked beautifully. Joanna then succeeded in breast-feeding both twins simultaneously for several months.

Conclusion: Alicia's ability to breast-feed was not affected by the fact that she had had seven whole weeks of bottle-feeding.*

Before your milk comes in

These first two or three days when your baby is getting your colostrum are probably the most important in terms of establishing breast-feeding. If you get your feeding technique right at this stage, breast-feeding will tend to go smoothly and you will be unlikely to develop any problems. But if you don't get it right, you will usually find that your feeds are unnecessarily long, you may well develop sore nipples and this could in turn be followed by engorged breasts and mastitis. I paint this gloomy picture to emphasise the point that most of these problems are caused by **poor attachment of the baby to the breast** – they are *not* part and parcel of breast-feeding.

It is therefore important to be aware of the following:

- It is usually harder for a baby to extract colostrum than it is for him to extract milk – this means that correct latching at every feed is particularly important in the first few days.
- There is not much colostrum in your breasts, so you should expect feeds to be relatively short – ideally lasting less than half an hour.
- If your baby wants to feed for a great deal longer than this, he is unlikely to be an exceptionally hungry baby. It is much more likely that he is not latched on correctly and is therefore not getting the colostrum as quickly and easily as he should.
- If your baby is doing long feeds (because he is latched on badly) you will almost certainly develop sore nipples within the first day or two.
- A baby that has fed well will usually stop feeding of his own accord and will settle well when you put him back in his cot.
- If your baby does not settle well after a feed, he is almost certainly still hungry.
- You should use both breasts at each feed, as there is no such thing as fore and hind colostrum. It is only when your milk comes in that you need to worry about foremilk and hindmilk, and start making decisions about whether you need to use one breast or two.

If your baby is latching on correctly and feeding well, you should be able to 'feed on demand' as he will give you clear signs as to when he needs feeding and when he has finished feeding. You would expect him to cry when he's hungry, feed reasonably quickly and then fall into a contented sleep when he's had enough. If he has taken a good feed, he should also last at least one hour (but preferably two to three hours) before he will ask to be fed again. If your baby is doing all of this you can relax and be fairly certain that all will continue to go well.

But if your baby is not latched on well you can expect him to want to feed a lot longer and a lot more frequently than this and he may well never settle into a contented sleep. If this happens, you must keep asking midwives to check your latching technique, otherwise you are almost certain to develop sore nipples and your baby will continue to struggle to get enough colostrum for his needs. This is not good either for you or for your baby and you will both end up tired and unhappy.

You should also note the following factors relating to long feeds:

● Not all babies stop sucking when they have had enough milk. You only have to see a baby happily sucking on a dummy or his mother's finger to realise that babies love sucking. It therefore seems logical to accept that a baby might sometimes continue sucking on his mother's breast for pleasure, rather than because he wants or needs more milk.

● Having seen literally hundreds of mothers with sore nipples, I have come to the conclusion that some do have more delicate nipples than others. These women are therefore at a greater risk of getting sore – in the same way that fair-skinned people will burn more easily in the sun. As a mother won't know whether she has particularly delicate nipples until she gets sore (by which time it's too late!), I think it is sensible to treat every one as being potentially at risk of becoming sore. The longer the feeds, the more likely she is to get sore.

● If you are very careful not to overdo feeding initially, you are unlikely to be suffering from sore nipples when your milk comes in – it is at this point that most babies become really hungry and you certainly don't want to be so sore that you can't feed.

Note: There is nearly always enough colostrum to keep even the largest baby satisfied until the milk comes in. However, if your baby constantly cries and appears hungry, and will not settle even after reasonably long and frequent feeds, you might need to give him some formula milk to tide him over until your milk comes in. Giving extra milk at this point is unlikely to have any detrimental effect on breast-feeding (e.g. by causing nipple–teat confusion) but should only be given as a last resort and preferably only on the advice of a midwife or paediatrician. It is, however, important to realise that the main reason a baby would need extra milk is that he is incorrectly positioned at the breast and, unless you can improve his latch, he will continue to get too little milk, even when your milk comes in.

When your milk comes in

You will know your milk is coming in when your breasts start becoming fuller and firmer. You may also notice the colour of your milk is changing from the yellow of colostrum to the paler colour of milk. If you are unlucky, you may temporarily suffer from engorged breasts but this is less likely to happen if you are feeding your baby at least every three to four hours at this stage. If you do get engorged breasts, refer to the section on Primary engorgement (page 113).

Feed regularly

As soon as your milk comes in it becomes essential that your breasts are emptied regularly throughout the day and night in order to keep the supply going. You would normally expect your baby to need to feed at least every three to four hours, thus having anything from six to nine feeds a day. If he is regularly taking more than nine feeds a day, it will make both of you very tired. Instead, try to get him to take bigger feeds, so that he needs feeding less often.

Frequency of feeds

- Try not to feed your baby more frequently than every two hours (timed from the start of one feed to the start of the next).
- Try to feed him at least every four hours during the day, even if it means waking him. If you feed him less frequently than this, he will almost certainly feed a lot more during the night to make up for his low milk intake during the day.
- If your baby sleeps soundly at night you can let him go as long as

he wants in between feeds, i.e. it is fine to let him go for much longer than four hours at night without a feed, provided he has had plenty of feeds during the day.

Note: If you are advised to feed your baby more frequently for medical reasons (e.g. if he is jaundiced) you should, of course, follow that advice.

Don't miss any feeds

At the stage when you are trying both to establish and maintain a good milk supply, it is not a good idea to miss out any feeds (e.g. in the middle of the night) because this will confuse your breasts and is likely to result in a reduction of milk. If you are absolutely exhausted, you could *occasionally* substitute a night-time breast-feed with a bottle but the more you do this the more detrimental it will be to your milk supply.

Note: If you miss out a night feed, and then wake in the morning with very full breasts, this is *not* a good sign. When this happens, many mothers assume that the missed feed has allowed their breasts time to fill up and that their milk supply during the day will be better as a result. However, what actually happens is that, as soon as the breasts become much fuller than usual, they get the message that they are overproducing milk and they may start reducing (rather than increasing) the amount they produce.

Expressing milk

When your milk first comes in, you might find that you have more than your baby needs. Although you do not want to over-stimulate your breasts (and thereby increase production), this is a good opportunity for you to express some of the surplus milk, which can then be kept in the freezer as a back-up for any time in the future when you might need it. Another reason for expressing at this stage is that many babies can be quite sleepy for the first week or so (especially if they are jaundiced), resulting in them taking less milk than they actually need. This can then be followed by a sudden increase in demand from the baby, which the breast is unable to meet, having been lulled into a false sense of security by the smaller feeds of the previous few days. If you have been expressing, you will have maintained a good supply of milk to cope with your baby's increased appetite.

Any milk you express can be kept in the fridge in a sterile bottle for up to 48 hours or frozen in special freezer bags (you can buy these from a chemist) for approximately three months. Milk which is not used within this time should be thrown away.

5 Coming home from hospital

Leaving hospital normally involves a mixture of emotions. Most mothers will be longing to get home to the comfort of their own bed and to have a night of sleep undisturbed by the crying of babies belonging to other mothers. This desire to get home is usually coupled with a fear of the unknown and worry about whether you will be able to cope on your own without the back-up of midwives being permanently on hand to offer advice and reassurance.

It will make a huge difference to your confidence if you have someone (e.g. your husband, mother or a maternity nurse) to stay with you for the first two weeks or so, until you have settled in with your new baby. Although you might still feel nervous, you will without doubt find the presence of someone else in the house very comforting and reassuring.

Rest

Giving birth is tiring for you and your baby and you will both need time to recover. In the past, mothers stayed in hospital for up to 10 days after their babies were born, during which time there was no question of them getting dressed, doing housework, preparing meals, or doing any entertaining. This allowed mothers time to recover from the birth and to get feeding established long before they returned to the isolation of their home. Unfortunately, this luxury is now no longer available as most hospitals expect you to leave within a day or two of giving birth. Many mothers even leave within a matter of hours.

You will, however, find that it will get you off to a really good start if you can try to follow the old-fashioned concept of 'lying-in'. This means spending the first 10 days after the birth mainly in bed, and certainly staying in your nightie rather than rushing around the house like a mad thing tidying up and checking what has been going on in your absence! At least once a day you should take the phone off the hook and attempt to have an uninterrupted sleep for an hour or so.

Time spent in catching up on your sleep during these first few days is time well spent. If you rush around too much you may find that not only do you become increasingly tired, but your milk supply may suffer as well. I think that many mothers become tearful and experience the 'baby blues' on or around Day 4, as much from tiredness as from hormonal changes that are beyond their control.

Visitors

It is tempting to be so proud of your new baby that you allow everyone who rings to come and visit you. This is a big mistake! The excitement will soon wear off and having too many visitors will not only make you very tired, but will also disrupt your routine with the baby with the result that he may not be fed when he needs to feed, or be left to sleep when he needs to sleep. A baby that is overtired or overhungry will soon become very unsettled and you may set the trend for disruptive days and nights.

Visitors should be monitored carefully and kept to a minimum. Of course, you will want family and close friends to come and see your baby, but it is a good idea to agree with your husband in advance how long you want them to stay. He can then be the one to ask them to leave if they are staying too long. Many visitors think that they should stay a long time in order to show sufficient interest in the new baby, so it is helpful for them (as well as you), to know how long the visit should last. Everyone knows that new mothers are lacking in sleep and need as much rest as they can get, so you are unlikely to cause any offence.

Cot death – safety for baby

I wasn't quite sure where in the book I should raise the issue of cot death, but eventually I decided that I should discuss it sooner rather than later. This is because I know that it is a major source of concern for new parents, and many of them start worrying about it almost as soon as they get home. The incidence of cot death dropped dramatically with the 'back to sleep' campaign and research continues to throw more light on the subject, with advice often changing as a result. For example, several childcare specialists have made a great point of recommending co-sleeping, but recent research has now shown that it is *not* advisable to have your baby sleeping in bed with you. I can therefore only give out the most recent information that is currently available, but would advise all new mothers to keep up to date with any new material that is published.

It is currently recommended that:

- The safest place for a baby to sleep is in a cot in the parents' bedroom for the first six months.
- A baby is laid on his back to sleep, *not* on his tummy.
- Your baby's head is left uncovered in his cot. You should lie him down with his feet touching the end of the cot – to prevent him slipping under the blankets.
- You do not let anyone smoke near your baby.
- Parents who smoke *anywhere* in the house put their baby at a greater risk than non-smokers.
- You should not let your baby get too hot.
- You do not let your baby sleep in bed with you, especially if you smoke, have been drinking alcohol or taking medications that make you sleepy.
- You should not feed your baby in bed if you are so tired that you might fall asleep.
- You should not sleep with your baby on a sofa or armchair.

If you can follow all the above suggestions, your baby will be receiving the best possible care and you should therefore try not to become too anxious about anything untoward happening to your baby.

Where your baby should sleep

There are many different views as to where a baby should sleep in the first few weeks. Although research (as mentioned above) has shown that it is best to put a baby to sleep in a separate cot, some childcare experts continue to disagree with this – they think that co-sleeping with your baby is an important part of mother–baby bonding, that it promotes breast-feeding and that it *is* safe. They say that a baby needs to remain close to his mother in order to feel secure and loved, and that it is wrong to deprive him of this comfort.

I completely disagree! I think every mother needs to appreciate that a normal healthy baby, who has had all his needs met, will sleep soundly and happily wherever you put him. If you look at a baby asleep in his cot, there is nothing to suggest that he is lying there thinking how mean and unloving his mother is – he is asleep and contented and totally unaware of where he is in relation to his mother. If, however, he does *not* fall sound asleep in his cot, the most likely reason will be that you have *not* met all his needs and you need to find out what the problem is and sort it. If you take him into bed with you without addressing the problem (e.g. hunger, wind) you will probably succeed in stopping him crying, but this is not the best way to resolve the issue.

I say this because:

- If a baby is still hungry or needs winding, all you have to do is meet these needs and he will happily go to sleep.
- If you can never find a way to stop him crying other than to cuddle him, you should consult a health professional to see whether he has a medical problem (e.g. reflux) that needs treating.
- There is strong evidence to suggest that it is risky to sleep with your baby.
- If your baby becomes accustomed to sleeping with you, this will almost certainly prove to be a hard habit to break when you eventually decide that you want him to sleep in his own bed.

The next issue is whether your baby should sleep in the same room as you or in his own room. From a safety point of view, you cannot go wrong having him in with you, but this may not suit all parents for a number of reasons:

- If you are a light sleeper, having him in your bedroom is likely to disturb your sleep unnecessarily, as you will wake with all his little baby noises rather than only being woken when he actually needs attention.
- If you are a noisy sleeper, you might find that you are waking your baby, rather than him waking you!
- Having your baby in your bedroom will result in both you *and* your husband being woken at feed times. This is fine if your husband wants to be fully involved, but if he has to go to work in the

morning, it seems a bit unnecessary to have both of you suffering from a lack of sleep. You at least should be able to catch up on lost sleep with a daytime nap.

If you do decide to put your baby in a separate room, the most important thing is that your baby should be within earshot – if he is too far away for you to hear him easily, you can always use a baby monitor.

During the day, your baby can sleep anywhere that suits you, but it is a good idea to keep him somewhere near you so that you can keep an eye on him and so that he gets used to sleeping through normal everyday noises – during the first few weeks, he shouldn't need quiet or darkness to keep him asleep. If you always tuck your baby away in an upstairs bedroom and creep around whenever he is sleeping, he will become used to total silence and will then tend to wake every time the phone rings, a doorbell goes or any other unexpected noise happens.

It may also help your baby to distinguish between night and day if, right from the start, you only put him to sleep in his bedroom at night. However, once you notice that he *is* beginning to become a bit more sensitive to noise, you will probably find that he will sleep longer and better during his naps if you put him to sleep in his bedroom with the curtains drawn. This usually happens after about three months.

Note: Babies tend to sleep longer and better when they are lying flat than they do when sitting up in a baby seat. For this reason you will probably find that it will make your life much more peaceful if you can get into the habit of putting him to sleep in his Moses basket, rather than continually leaving him to cat nap in his bouncing chair. Whenever possible, you should also transfer him back into his Moses basket (or crib or pram) after a journey, rather than leaving him in his car seat. Of course, if you find that doing this always wakes your baby and he is then unable to settle back to sleep in his Moses basket, it is better to leave him sleeping in his car seat.

Room temperature

When you take your baby home your house will need to be warmer than usual but not as hot as it was in hospital.

A house temperature of about 20°C (68°F) will be warm enough for your baby. You can keep your house cooler than this (it won't harm him), but it might seem rather chilly when you are breast-feeding. It may also be a bit too cold for your baby when you are changing his nappy, bathing him, etc. However, I notice that a lot of mothers nowadays are obsessive about room temperature, to the extent of keeping a thermometer on their baby's cot, and then panicking if the temperature varies by a degree or two. It is absolutely pointless to be this precise unless you also know exactly how many clothes your baby should be wearing at each point of the temperature gauge. It is far better to be guided by common sense, which will tell you to put more clothes on him when he is in a cold place and take some off when he is in a warm place.

Your baby is not as fragile as you might think and will come to no harm if he is slightly too warm or slightly too cold. He will only be at risk if you get it so completely wrong that he is far too hot or freezing cold.

The best way to judge whether you are getting it right is to dress him in as many clothes as seems sensible and then check his body temperature when he wakes up for his next feed. It is normal for his hands and feet to feel a bit chilly, but the rest of his body should feel warm to the touch. If your baby's body is pleasantly warm but his hands and feet are cold, the sensible thing to do is to use mittens and bootees rather than piling on extra clothes and blankets.

During the winter months you will need to make sure that his room does not get too cold at night when the central heating goes off – cold is a common cause of a baby waking at night, especially as he gets older and starts wriggling out from under his blankets. The most economical way to keep your baby's room warm is to use a convector heater or an electric radiator with thermostatic controls. Remember, your baby will get cold more quickly than you will, partly because he is so small and partly because he is not generating heat by moving around as an adult does.

Note: Whenever I come across a particularly anxious mother, who is still worrying about whether her house is too warm or too cold, I ask her this question: Are you ever planning to take your baby out of your house, and if so, will you only venture forth if the temperature outside is exactly the same as it is indoors? Common sense is all that is required!

Help in the home

It makes a big difference to a new mother to have some help and company once she gets home. Many partners will take the first week off work and be there to help with the cooking, shopping and nappy-changing and other baby-related things. Nowadays most men are pretty helpful around the house, are keen to get involved with the care of their newborn baby and can be a great source of support and comfort to their wives.

If you are on your own or your husband cannot be at home with you, it is ideal if your mother can come and help, either right from the outset or to take over when/if your husband has to go back to work. It's helpful to remember that your mother looked after you when you were a baby and, although you might think that her views will be out of date, you may be surprised to find that a lot of her advice actually works! There is nothing like age and experience when it comes to dealing with babies.

You will almost certainly find your mother's presence very reassuring, and it will also be nice for you to have company during the day and to have someone to 'mother' and look after you by preparing meals and looking after your baby while you have an afternoon sleep.

I well remember going to stay with my parents when my first baby was only a few weeks old. Even though I was a midwife, there were many occasions when my baby was crying and I didn't have a clue what to do! It was my mother who showed me how to settle my baby to sleep on my lap (when all other methods had failed) and it was also she who taught me that sometimes it is in the best interests of a baby to be left to cry himself to sleep. Without my mother's help and advice in those early weeks, I think I would have been a nervous wreck and would have missed out on learning what I now consider to be fairly essential parenting skills. Granny sometimes knows best!

Maternity nurses

If you decide to employ a maternity nurse you will usually find that personal recommendations are the most reliable way of finding a good one. Using a reputable nanny agency is your next best option as the agency will normally check the references of any maternity nurse they supply. Scanning magazine ads is a much more hit-and-miss affair than going through personal recommendations or an agency, although it is still possible to get a good maternity nurse this way.

Before booking a maternity nurse, interview her carefully to try and establish whether her views reflect your own. It is also helpful to establish in advance exactly what her duties will be. Some maternity nurses will only do things that directly involve the baby, while others are willing to do anything that will make your life easier, e.g. helping with the cooking and making cups of tea for you and your visitors.

You will also need to find out how flexible your maternity nurse can be in terms of her starting date. Babies are rarely born exactly on their due date and it would be a shame to book a nurse for a month and then find that for the first two weeks your baby has not even put in an appearance! If in doubt, it's probably better to book her for approximately two weeks after your due date (first babies are usually born later, rather than earlier than expected), on the basis that you can probably survive initially with the help of your husband or mother.

A good and experienced maternity nurse should:

- Teach you how to do everything involved in the care of a newborn baby. Even the simplest of things such as knowing how many clothes to put on your baby can be worrying to a new mother. Gaining confidence in these matters in the early days will set you up well for the future.
- Help you to learn to differentiate between your baby's various cries, i.e. help you get to know whether your baby is crying because he is hungry or needs winding, or because he is overtired, etc.
- Help you to establish breast-feeding (and/or bottle-feeding), guiding you as to how long and how often to feed.
- Discourage you, your friends and your family from making your baby overtired and overstimulated by playing with him too much in between feeds. In the early days, your baby needs to be left to sleep in peace.
- Help to guide (but not force) your baby into a good feeding and sleeping pattern.
- Help you to rest and recover from the birth by doing most of the time-consuming things involved with a new baby, i.e. nappy changing, winding and settling after feeds. The latter in particular will make a huge difference to your night-time feeds.
- Bring your baby into your bedroom at night only when he needs to feed, enabling you to get as much sleep as possible.
- Boost your confidence by making you feel that you are a competent mother, so that you don't panic when she leaves!

Your maternity nurse should not:

- Force your baby into a strict and inflexible feeding routine. Although I am all in favour of aiming towards a good routine, it is not fair on the baby to be too strict in the early weeks, nor does it help with establishing a good milk supply.
- Be bossy and insist that everything be done her way or not at all! She can (and should) advise you as to what should be done but ultimately most, if not all, decisions concerning your baby should be made by you and your husband.
- Hog your baby and refuse to allow you and your husband to have *any* access to him in between feeds, on the basis that you will disrupt her routine with the baby. Unfortunately, some maternity nurses are inclined to do this.
- Undermine your confidence by continually disagreeing with you, the district midwife, health visitor, etc.

Doulas

Doulas can be hired in much the same way as a maternity nurse and are proving to be an increasingly popular choice for mothers. A doula is an experienced woman who has been trained to provide both practical and emotional support for the whole family after the birth. Her hours are flexible and you can arrange with her how often you want her to come in, for how many hours she stays and for how many weeks she continues to visit. You can expect her to help with household chores, shopping, cooking, breast-feeding support and practical help with the baby and any other children. In other words, she will normally do everything your own mother would do!

District midwives

Under the present law, all mothers and babies must be seen by a midwife for the first 10 days after the birth, after which time she hands over to a health visitor. Ideally, a midwife should visit every day but if she has a very large workload she may only visit you every other day, provided all is well with you both. However, if you want or need her to visit more often than this, she will usually be happy to do so.

The district midwife's role is to check your health and make sure that your uterus is contracting back down after the birth. She will also check your baby and do the routine tests that are always carried out in the first 10 days. She will weigh your baby and advise you what to do if you are having feeding or any other problems and, if she thinks it necessary, she may carry on visiting you beyond Day 10.

Health visitor

Your health visitor will usually call by, on or around Day 10. She will give you a booklet in which to keep records of your baby's development, weight, etc. She will also tell you where your nearest baby clinic is and how to get hold of her should you need her. She is the one who will be giving you more general advice on baby care. She will check that your baby is reaching his milestones and will also tell you when he needs his injections, hearing tests, etc.

Most health visitors are absolutely excellent, but occasionally you might be unlucky and come across one who will inadvertently demoralise and upset you. This tends to happen when the health visitor is too keen to go exactly 'by the book' when it comes to things like weight gain, rather than having the confidence to use her own judgement to see whether the baby is thriving and healthy. I have had many mothers over the years ring me in floods of tears because their health visitor has got them in a panic (worrying that they have damaged their baby) simply because the baby has gained an ounce or two less than the charts show he should have. Of course, it is important to keep an eye on your baby's weight gain but it will take more than a few ounces here and there to damage him. If you are worried about your baby you can always visit your GP or a paediatrician and get their opinion.

6 General feeding advice

Even when breast-feeding is going really well, many a mother will still worry about whether she is doing everything right. And if she asks questions, a mother may find that everyone tells her something different, and it can be hard to know whose advice to follow. This chapter covers all the common questions that I have been asked over the years and, where appropriate, gives the different views that might be expressed on the subject.

Feeding twins

There is absolutely no reason why a mother should be unable to breast-feed twins as most breasts are perfectly capable of producing enough milk to feed two babies. Many mothers find it very easy and have no problems at all, either in latching them on simultaneously or in producing plenty of milk for them both.

However, some mothers find that coping with twins is very tiring and difficult, and that, despite their best efforts, they are unable to produce enough milk for two babies. I think that any mother with twins should be realistic and recognise that she *will* find it harder to cope with two babies, and that she is not a failure if she is unable to breast-feed both fully. Twins that cannot get enough milk from the breast are usually perfectly happy to take a mixture of breast milk and formula milk, so being unable to produce plenty of breast milk doesn't mean giving up breast-feeding completely.

It is particularly important to take care of yourself when feeding twins. Don't neglect your own needs for food and rest, and try to put everything else you want to do on hold until you have got breast-feeding well established. Time spent establishing your milk supply in the first few weeks may well set you up for many months of breast-feeding, so it's worth investing plenty of time and effort from the beginning. If possible, arrange to have someone to help you in the early weeks as it can be quite difficult to cope with two babies when it comes to latching on, winding, etc. Although some mothers manage amazingly well right from the word go, they are the exception, so don't feel demoralised if you can't manage on your own.

Ideally, you should aim to breast-feed twins simultaneously, as this will allow you some respite in between feeds. However, this can be easier said than done. Just as some mothers find it hard to latch on one baby (especially if their nipples are not the ideal shape), mothers of twins can experience the same problem twofold. If you do have problems latching on the babies, it's better to start off feeding one at a time in the conventional way (so that you can concentrate fully on each baby) and then try to graduate on to feeding them simultaneously as you all become more experienced.

The easiest way to feed twins simultaneously is to use the 'football hold' (see page 43) and to sit in bed or on a sofa (rather than on a chair) so that you can use plenty of pillows and cushions to support the babies. If you are particularly skilful you may be able to hold a baby in each hand and latch each one on without needing an extra hand to shape your breast. Much more commonly, however, you will need to concentrate on getting one baby latched on properly before being handed the second (by your helper) and repeating the process. Once the babies are latched on, you can allow them to stay on the same breast for the whole feed (rather than swapping breasts at the halfway stage) and only take them off to wind them as and when necessary. It's a good idea to alternate the breast each baby has at subsequent feeds as it is highly likely that one baby will feed a bit better than the other, and as a result, will do a better job of emptying the breast. By alternating breasts you will be able to ensure that each breast gets fully stimulated (by the baby who feeds the best) for at least half of the feeds.

If you have plenty of milk you should find that the babies settle well after feeds and gain the right amount of weight. If you are not producing enough milk you will probably find that each feed takes a minimum of one hour and the babies will then either not settle at all, or will only doze off to sleep for a short time before waking up again, wanting more food.

If this happens you have three choices:

1. You can try to improve your milk supply (see page 126).
2. You can give both babies top-up bottles (of expressed or formula milk) at the end of any feed when they are still hungry.
3. You can breast-feed one baby (using both breasts) while the other is given a bottle of formula milk and then reverse the process at the next feed so that each baby gets a turn at the breast. You can carry on doing this for as long as it suits you all.

Note: Most twins are delivered earlier than their due date and are likely to be smaller (and possibly slightly weaker) than a full-term single baby. As a result, some twins are not able to breast-feed initially and may need to be given some or all of their feeds by bottle. If this happens, you should express milk every three to four hours (during the night as well as during the day), partly to stimulate and maintain your milk supply and partly to enable your babies to be given expressed breast milk rather than formula. Don't worry that this will stop your babies breast-feeding at a later date – most babies happily transfer to the breast as soon as they are strong enough.

As it is common for one twin to be a better feeder than the other (and therefore to take bigger feeds which satisfy him for longer), it may not always be possible to establish a routine whereby they are both fed at the same time. If you can synchronise them, all to the good, but you will need to decide whether it's worth the effort and whether it's in the best interests of the babies if one twin is clearly less able to go as long in between feeds as the other. However, it is usually possible to get the babies synchronised at some stage, even if you can't manage it in the early weeks.

Hygiene
There is always a risk of cross-infection between twins, so it is important to be meticulous about hygiene, treating each baby as an individual. This doesn't mean that you always have to wash your hands in between handling one baby and the other, say, during feed times, but you should wash your hands in between nappy changes, preparing bottles, etc., in the same way as you would if you only had one baby.

The babies should not suck from the same bottle or share a dummy, but they can share your breasts! However, if one has an infection (e.g. thrush in his mouth) you would be well advised to wash your breast very thoroughly after he has fed and you should also wash your hands carefully every time you handle that baby.

Most twins like to be physically close to each other and will usually settle better if they are put to sleep in the same cot, but if one of them develops an infection or a minor illness such as a cold, it makes sense to keep them apart until the ill one is better. It is also worth separating them if one twin keeps being disturbed and woken by the other, as there is no point having two wakeful babies!

Drugs and breast-feeding

Most over-the-counter drugs such as paracetamol are safe to take while breast-feeding, but it is good practice always to read the literature that comes with any medication, to check whether it is contra-indicated for breast-feeding mothers.

If your GP prescribes any medicine for you, it is worth reminding him that you are breast-feeding (even if the prescription is for mastitis!) as all GPs are human and can easily forget to take this into consideration when deciding which drug to prescribe.

Note: Some drugs (e.g. antibiotics) may well have an adverse effect on your baby and temporarily give him diarrhoea or make him uncomfortable with wind or colic. So long as his symptoms are relatively mild and stop once you have finished the course of drugs, there is no cause for concern. If however, your baby reacts very badly, you should certainly consult your doctor or local pharmacist.

Breast surgery

A mother who has had a breast reduction is fairly unlikely to be able to breast-feed because the milk ducts are disconnected in the surgical process. But a mother who has had other breast surgery (e.g. to excise benign or malignant growths, or breast enhancement) will probably have been told by her surgeon that she should still be able to breast-feed, although he will not be able to give her an absolute guarantee on this. I have known mothers who have successfully breast-fed following breast surgery and others who have been unable to establish breast-feeding. As it is impossible to predict in advance how breast surgery will affect individual women, I would advise all mothers to give breast-feeding a try, but not to feel a failure if it doesn't work out for them.

Note: I recently visited a mother who had previously had surgery to remove a lump from one of her breasts. Her unaffected breast was working perfectly, but the one that had been operated on was becoming extremely engorged, lumpy and uncomfortable, and no milk was coming out. We eventually managed to extract a small amount by hand-expressing but we were unable to get her milk flowing properly. After several days her breast stopped producing milk and eventually softened up and returned to normal. Her 'good' breast continued to work well so she was able to carry on breast-feeding and supplement with formula milk whenever necessary.

Weight gain

Your baby's weight gain is the best indication as to whether or not he is getting enough food and is developing as he should. Having said this, not all babies follow the charts exactly as they should, but this does not necessarily mean that they are not perfectly healthy and thriving. The most important thing to bear in mind is that babies are individuals and should be treated as such, but if you are concerned about your baby's development it is far better to consult a doctor or paediatrician than to sit at home worrying.

When weighing your baby, you will need to take the following factors into account, especially if he is gaining less weight than expected:

● His birth weight may have been inaccurately measured or recorded and this will reflect on his subsequent weight measurements.
● A baby's weight at birth is usually affected by a combination of maternal diet and placental function, and does not necessarily reflect the size he will end up, i.e. a baby born to small parents (but whose mother ate well during her pregnancy and had an efficient placenta) could start off being quite large but is then likely, at some stage, to slow his growth so that eventually he will end up a similar size to his parents. This will result in a slowing of weight gain at some point in his development and is both normal and expected.
● By the same token, a small baby born to large parents will almost certainly have a growth spurt at some stage, resulting in his temporarily putting on more weight than the charts indicate he should.
● Scales are not always accurate, especially if different ones are

used each time your baby is weighed, so don't panic if he doesn't appear to gain exactly the right amount of weight one week.

● It's best to weigh a normal baby (i.e. a full-term, healthy baby) no more frequently than once a week (after Day 10). This is because a baby's weight can fluctuate quite a bit each day depending on whether you weigh him before or after a feed, or before or after a wet nappy. For example, a baby who is weighed straight after a 90 ml (3 oz) feed, will weigh 90 g (3 oz) more than he would if he had been weighed immediately before the feed.

Your baby will be weighed as soon as he is born and then fairly frequently (usually every other day) until he is 10 days old. This will be done by the midwives in hospital, and by the district midwife who will bring scales with her when she visits you at home. Your health visitor will come and see you about 10 days after your baby is born and she will give you a Child Health Record which you keep at home and use to keep notes of your baby's development, weight gain, etc. It has charts at the back for recording his head circumference, length and weight so you can see for yourself whether he is putting on the right amount of weight.

A baby will normally lose about 10 per cent of his birth weight in the first few days (this is both normal and expected), then start putting on weight again from about Day 4 or 5 and get back to his birth weight sometime between Days 10–14. From then on, he should gain approximately 150–210 g (5–7 oz) a week until he's about three months old. Some babies have a very variable weight gain, sometimes gaining, say, only 120 g (4 oz) one week and then as much as 300–360 g (10–12 oz) the next week. With this in mind, you shouldn't panic if your baby's weight gain is uneven and should look more at his general signs of contentment and overall weight gain, i.e. whether he is at the approximate weight he should be at any one time. You will be able to plot his weight on the chart every time you weigh him.

Although it is important that your baby gains weight fairly steadily, it will rarely do him any harm to go a week or two gaining slightly more or less weight than he should. However, if either you or your health visitor are worried about his weight gain it may be a good idea to take him to a doctor and get him checked over. The doctor will then be able to advise you as to what, if anything, you need to do. (An indication that your baby is underfed is if his stools become slightly green as opposed to mustard-yellow.)

Note: Some babies gain far more weight than the charts indicate they should. Provided you aren't continually feeding your baby at times when he is crying for reasons other than hunger (e.g. tiredness or boredom), there is little that you can do about it. It is very normal for some babies to consume vast quantities of milk (regardless of whether they are breast-feeding or bottle-feeding) and it is extremely hard to restrict the amount of milk that you need to give to keep such hungry babies contented in between feeds. If you are bottle-feeding you could try changing to a formula milk for the hungrier baby (to see whether this satisfies him better), but ultimately you need to relax and give him as much milk as he needs and not worry about his excessive weight gain. You will usually find that a baby like this will need to start on solids before the recommended six months – you can discuss this with your health visitor. Once your baby is having some solid food he will almost certainly become more contented, his milk consumption will go down and his weight gain will usually slow down as well.

How much milk does your baby need?

As a very rough guide, most babies under the age of four months will need approximately 150 ml of milk per kg of body weight (or 2½–3oz per 1 lb), during each 24-hour period. The amount of milk a baby takes at each feed will depend on how many feeds he is having a day and will also vary a bit from feed to feed, according to his appetite. For example:

Metric

For a 3 kg baby on six feeds a day, you would multiply 3 kg by 150 ml = 450 ml. Divided by six feeds = 75 ml per feed.

Imperial

For a 7 lb baby on seven feeds a day, you would multiply 7 lb by 3 oz = 21 oz. Divided by seven feeds = 3 oz per feed. (For ease of maths, I have multiplied by 3 oz, rather than by 2½ oz).

This is only a rough guide so don't worry if your baby is taking slightly more or less than this – as long as his weight gain is good you will be getting it right.

What about extra water?

Neither a breast-fed nor a bottle-fed baby should need any extra water as milk provides all the fluid he will need. However, if the weather is particularly hot and you feel your baby may be thirsty as opposed to hungry, you could try offering him extra, cool boiled water in between feeds. You can also give water in between feeds to an unsettled baby as a way of keeping him going until a feed is due, in much the same way as you might give an apple to a grizzling toddler. It can help to offer extra water to a baby who is constipated, although a baby who is fully breast-fed rarely suffers from constipation.

Note: Be careful not to give so much water that your baby is then too full to take his milk feed. There are no calories in water, so you shouldn't give him water if he is hungry or if his weight gain is poor.

How long should a feed last?

The answer is: long enough for your baby to get enough milk to last him until the next feed – which ideally would be about three to four hours later. It is very important to make this point, because so many mothers are now told to 'feed on demand' without being given any guidelines as to what the average baby actually needs.

So, the basic fact to keep in mind is this – a normal healthy baby, when offered enough milk, will normally choose to feed roughly every three to four hours and have between six and nine feeds in each 24-hour period. If your baby *regularly* wants to feed much more than this, you are almost certainly trying to settle him down when he has only had a snack, rather than a proper meal. In fact, feeding your baby is fairly similar to feeding a toddler – if you make sure that he eats a proper lunch, he shouldn't need any more food until teatime. But if he doesn't eat enough lunch, he will almost certainly want to snack all afternoon and then he won't be hungry enough to eat his next meal properly. And so it goes on...

When discussing how long a feed should last it is important to differentiate between how long you spend involved with a feed (i.e. from the baby waking to the baby going back to sleep) and how long the baby is actually feeding. When I refer to a feed I am talking about the actual time spent feeding rather than nappy-changing, winding, etc.

The length of your feeds will depend on how strongly your baby sucks, how well he is latched on to the breast, how fast your milk is released (see The let-down reflex, page 17) and also how much milk you have. An average-length feed would last approximately 20 minutes, a slow feed can take anything up to an hour and a fast feed can be over in 10 minutes or less. With this in mind, you need to find out how long it takes *your* baby to get enough milk out of *your* breasts to last him three to four hours.

To do this, you should:

- Start feeding your baby when he is clearly hungry.
- Keep him feeding on the first breast until he stops sucking effectively (i.e. when his sucks become shallow and infrequent), which would indicate that your breast is nearly or even completely empty.
- Offer him the second breast and allow him to feed on that as above.
- When he no longer wants to feed on the second breast, you can hope that this means he is full, rather than your breast is empty
- Settle him down to sleep and see what happens.
- Make a note (for future reference) of how long he spent on each breast.

If your baby settles well and doesn't need feeding again for a reasonable length of time (i.e. approximately three to four hours, timed from the start of the previous feed) you will know that you got it right and you can hope that the next feed will follow a similar pattern. But if he *doesn't* settle well every time you follow his cues (as above) it is time for you to take charge to persuade him to stay awake and feed a bit longer. You would do this by changing his nappy, taking some or even all of his clothes off and possibly by opening a nearby window. If these tactics work and he feeds for a few minutes longer and then settles better, you will have discovered how long *your* feeds need to last in order to give *your* baby a full feed.

As you will now realise, judging how long it takes your baby to get enough milk from your breast will take time as it is not something you can learn overnight – even an experienced midwife would find it difficult to judge accurately whether a baby has had enough milk by supervising only one feed. It is only by seeing how long your baby stays asleep between one feed and the next that you will know whether he had enough milk at the previous feed. As a result, one tends to be wise only after the event. However, timing (but not limiting) your feeds will help you to see a pattern emerge, and weighing your baby regularly will also reassure you as to whether you are feeding him enough.

Don't worry if you don't get it exactly right to begin with because your baby will come to no harm if he is occasionally fed slightly too little or slightly too much during the early days when you are both still at the learning stage.

Note: It is vital to the success of breast-feeding not to restrict the length of time your baby spends at the breast at any one feed. However, if your feeds regularly last much more than an hour, you should check to see whether your baby is latched on correctly (see page 102) because a baby that *is* latched on correctly will rarely need to spend more than an hour feeding. You should also check to see whether you have enough milk (see page 125).

Feeding on demand

Feeding on demand is crucial to the success of breast-feeding but in order to do this you need to understand what it means. Contrary to what many mothers think, it does not mean feeding your baby whenever he cries – it means feeding your baby whenever he cries *because he's hungry*. A baby will cry for all sorts of reasons and you need to try and find out *why* he is crying, rather than automatically assuming that he is hungry and immediately putting him to the breast.

A baby will cry if he is overtired, over-stimulated, uncomfortable with wind, colic or a dirty nappy, or simply when he is trying to go to sleep but can't because his mother keeps picking him up every time he cries! I am often called to visit a mother who is worried that she doesn't have enough milk because her baby is crying all day long and, no matter how long and how often she feeds him, he still won't settle. When I arrive I am regularly confronted by an exhausted mother *and* an exhausted baby, both of whom are in tears and desperate to get some sleep. It doesn't take long to establish that all the baby needs is to be wrapped up firmly and rocked to sleep, and this is what I do (see page 38).

It can be hard for a new mother to be able to judge whether it is sleep or food that he needs, especially when she finds that he will nearly always feed for a bit (even if he's not hungry) whenever she puts him to the breast. This leads her to believe that her baby must be hungry, whereas in fact he is probably just using her breast as a dummy and is sucking for comfort rather than from a desire to have more milk.

Many of the mothers I meet think that feeding on demand means that they should not attempt to initiate any kind of routine. They also think that they should always feed for as long and as often as their baby appears to want, even if it means spending most of the day (and night) feeding. The thinking behind this seems to be that a baby will only carry on sucking at the breast if he needs more milk and will then only wake again when he is hungry (and not for any other reason).

However, I would point out the following:

- A baby will suck on anything that you put in his mouth, so the fact that he might suck on your breast for hours on end does not necessarily mean that he is hungry, or even that he is getting any milk.
- A baby will wake and cry for all sorts of reasons, of which hunger is only one. If you always assume that it is hunger that's waking him you may end up feeding a baby who is crying with another problem (such as colic) which may be made worse if you feed him.
- If you feed your baby every time he is a bit peckish rather than waiting until he is genuinely hungry you will merely teach him to snack.
- It is hard for any mother to understand exactly what feeding on demand (using no guidelines) will involve until she actually does it. This is because it is not until your baby is born that you realise that feeding two-hourly, for example, does not mean that you do a quick feed and then have two hours of peace until the next feed. What it actually means is that, if your feeds take up to an hour, you may have a gap of only one hour between feeds. This would barely give you time to rest or grab something to eat before getting involved with the next feed. The problem with feeding this often is that it can make a mother so exhausted by the demands of her baby that her milk supply may dwindle rather than increase.
- In my experience, a baby that is fed three to four-hourly will usually start sleeping through the night sooner than a baby who is fed for weeks on end at totally random times, with his mother making no attempt to space out feeds.

Note: Feeds are timed from the point at which you *start* feeding (because a baby normally takes most of the milk at the beginning of the feed), rather than the point at which you finish.

To help you to know when to feed and when not to feed, I recommend the following:

1. *Try not to feed within two hours of the previous feed.*
Your baby is unlikely to be starving within two hours of the start of the previous feed, so if he cries within that time you should try to find out *why* he is crying rather than immediately assuming that he needs food. Instead of feeding him, first see if you can get him to go back to sleep by rocking him and patting his back gently as he lies (on his side) in his crib. You could also give him a dummy to suck on for comfort. If this doesn't settle him, you could pick him up to see whether he needs winding or a nappy change and then try putting him down to sleep again. If you do manage to get him back to sleep you will have learnt the valuable lesson that a crying baby does not always need feeding.

However, if nothing settles your baby and he won't stop crying, you should feed him because this would indicate that he *is* in fact hungry and it would be totally wrong simply to leave him crying and ignore his needs. It is perfectly normal for a baby occasionally to have unsettled periods, during which time all routine will go out the window while you muddle through, not really knowing what to do. Babies do not work like clockwork and sometimes you just have to go with the flow. But if your baby carries on being unsettled for too long (i.e. for more than 24 hours or so) you will need to go back to basics to try and re-establish a three to four-hourly routine (see The unsettled baby, page 137). This is because a baby that is regularly fed far too frequently will never be sufficiently hungry to take a proper feed and is therefore much more likely to have a snack which will then only last him another two hours or so. Another consequence of feeding too frequently is that it won't give your breasts the chance to fill up completely, which means they will be unlikely ever to have enough milk to give him a feed that will last him for four hours.

2. *Try to feed your baby at least every four hours during the day.*
During the first few weeks a baby will normally need at least six feeds

during each 24-hour period. Ideally, he should wake for these feeds on a fairly regular basis, e.g. approximately every three to four hours, but in practice this doesn't always happen. You may well find that your baby sleeps like a log during the day, going for at least five hours in between feeds, but that you then pay the price by having a much more disturbed night. This is because the less your baby feeds during the day, the more he will need to feed at night.

Your best chance of avoiding disturbed nights, therefore, is to ensure that your baby feeds reasonably often during the day – this is why I recommend that you try to feed him at least every four hours, even if it means waking him. If he is fairly easy to wake, feeds well, settles well and then sleeps well at night, you should continue to wake him during the day for his feeds. But if you find that waking him disrupts the day for both of you and he still wakes very frequently at night, then it is better to leave him to sort out his own feeding and sleeping patterns. You must then hope that he will start sleeping longer at night of his own accord.

If you can manage to stick to these simple guidelines you should find that your baby will settle into a very manageable feeding pattern and that your breasts get the right messages to ensure that they continue to produce plenty of milk.

Feeding on a strict four-hourly schedule (I do not recommend this)

In my experience mothers tend to fall into two main categories:

1. Those who are very relaxed and easy-going and who are perfectly prepared to feed their baby as and when he needs it, without worrying too much when he feeds and when he sleeps – i.e. they are happy to take life as it comes.
2. Those who like routine and order in their lives and who would like to get their babies feeding on a strict four-hourly schedule right from the word go.

I can sympathise with mothers in the second category because I know that I would have found motherhood much easier in the first few weeks had I been able (I wasn't!) to get each of my babies into a strict feeding routine from the outset. Unfortunately, babies aren't little machines that can be programmed to conform totally to their mother's wishes, and they will often become increasingly unhappy and unsettled if you force them into an unnatural (for them) feeding routine.

Although you can usually succeed in making a baby wait exactly four hours for a feed whenever he wakes too early (by holding him and rocking him, etc.) it is not a good idea to do this. This is because when you are breast-feeding it is impossible to know for sure exactly how much milk your baby has taken at any one feed. Your breasts may have given him only three hours' worth of milk and, if this is the case, you can't then expect him to last a full four hours until he is fed again. If you try to make him wait that extra hour for the feed, it's not only unkind to him, but it will also give your breasts the wrong message – i.e. it will make them think they have provided four hours' worth of milk. If you keep making your baby wait exactly four hours for each feed, he will become increasingly hungry and your breasts will continue to provide three hours' worth of milk, having never been given the message that they are providing too little.

Note: Even if you are bottle-feeding, you still cannot expect to slot your baby straight into a four-hourly routine. This is because a baby can only take the amount of milk that his stomach is capable of holding and there is no way of knowing whether your baby has the stomach capacity to hold four hours' worth of milk.

Because of these factors, it's really not a good idea to be too rigid about feeding schedules, although this doesn't mean that you have to abandon all hope of establishing a reasonable routine. What you can do is to attempt to get your baby into a good feeding pattern by making sure that he takes a proper feed each time (rather than just having a small snack), and then making sure that you don't feed him again until he is genuinely hungry. By doing this, you will give both of you the best chance of introducing some routine and order into your day.

Note: If you have a rather smug friend who tells you that she *did* manage to get her baby into a strict four-hourly routine from the outset, remember this – either she was very lucky and happened to have a baby who chose to adopt this routine (and some do) or it may be that her recollections are not strictly accurate!

Settling into a routine

For at least the first two or three weeks you are unlikely to establish any kind of a routine, other than trying not to feed your baby too often, i.e. preferably not more than nine times a day. But once your milk supply is well-established and you know there is plenty of milk for your baby, you can start trying to ease him into a better feeding pattern if he hasn't already got into one of his own accord. You will find it easier to know his needs by this time as you will probably be getting quite good at recognising when he is tired, hungry or needs winding.

From about three weeks onwards, your baby will hopefully rarely need feeding more frequently than every three hours and will sometimes go a good four hours in between feeds. As a general rule, he will automatically settle into this pattern if all his needs are being met and he is not suffering from any problem such as colic. But if your baby is not doing this, it would be quite wrong to force him into a strict routine overnight. You can, however, see whether you can persuade him to last a little bit longer in between feeds and if you can achieve this relatively easily (i.e. without changing your happy baby into a tearful, hungry one), all to the good. If, on the other hand, you find that he becomes unhappy and more unsettled when his feeding patterns are changed, it is best not to rock the boat and to leave him feeding as he was.

Suggestions that might improve feeding times
- Check whether your milk supply is good and try to increase it if it isn't (see page 125).
- Make sure you are feeding your baby for long enough at each feed and not letting him fall asleep before he has had enough milk.
- If your baby is suffering from excessive wind, colic or anything else that is making him uncomfortable, see your GP who may be able to prescribe something that will help.
- If you have a very 'sucky' baby who needs the comfort of something to suck on in between feeds, try using a dummy. Do **not** give a dummy to a baby who might be hungry – he needs food, not a dummy.
- Try offering water in between feeds – this may help settle him until a feed is due.

Note: You should not offer water if your milk supply is low and your baby is hungry. A hungry baby needs calories and filling him up with water instead of milk is not the answer – not only will this affect his appetite and deprive him of essential calories but it may also prevent him feeding enough at the breast to stimulate your milk supply.

Waking at 10pm?

From about six weeks onwards, it would be realistic to start hoping that your baby will sleep longer at night and that you may soon see the end of night feeds. Provided he is being given enough milk during the day, a baby will usually start sleeping through the night without you needing to do anything. However, some babies don't sleep through the night until they are at least three months old and others go on waking at night for a lot longer than this.

As a general rule, it works best to leave a baby to form his own sleep pattern at night and you should only try to change it if you are finding it totally unacceptable. For example, some mothers are thrilled if their baby starts sleeping through the 10pm feed, while others would prefer to carry on doing the 10pm feed and have the longest sleep time taking place after this. The main problem with trying to change your baby's natural sleep pattern is that you may make things worse rather than better.

As long as you are aware of this risk, you could try waking your baby for the 10pm feed and see what happens. If he feeds well, settles back to sleep quickly and then sleeps longer as a result, it may be worth continuing to wake him. But if you find that waking your baby upsets him and doesn't make any difference to how long he sleeps afterwards, it really would be better to leave him sleeping through the 10pm feed – this is clearly better for him, even if it is not better for you.

Night feeds

If you are breast-feeding, you really do need to do all the feeds including the ones at night, otherwise your breasts will get in a terrible muddle. Also, if you miss out a night feed, you may well find that you regret doing this if you then wake an hour or two later with very engorged, uncomfortable breasts.

If you're desperate to catch up on some sleep, it's probably fine to miss the occasional feed and let someone else give your baby a bottle, but ideally you would then express some extra milk during the day, both to keep your milk supply up and to provide your own milk (rather than formula) for the night feed. I do know of some mothers who never did the middle-of-the night feed and it had no adverse effect at all on their breast-feeding. But I have to say that I have seen many more mothers who had thought it was working quite well, and then gradually realised over a number of weeks that their milk supply was diminishing and they had to start giving complementary bottles during the day.

Either way, of course, the decision is yours, but it would be a shame to miss out too many night feeds and then find that it is affecting the rest of your breast-feeding. In theory, you should be able to increase your milk supply again if this happens (by feeding more often), but it can become quite an uphill battle and this is really best avoided.

Note: There is plenty of evidence to suggest that night feeds give a greater boost to milk production than daytime feeds – on this basis alone, I would urge mothers to bear this in mind when considering missing night feeds.

Dummies

People tend to have very strong opinions about dummies. They either love them or loathe them and rarely take a middle-of-the-road view on them.

Personally, I loathe them, but it didn't stop me from using one for both my children, nor has it stopped me from recommending them (when needed) to other mothers! This is because, while I find them extremely unattractive, I think that a dummy can be an invaluable aid when it comes to settling some babies. Although there is a theory that giving a baby a dummy will limit his intelligence, I would imagine that this would only apply when the dummy has been used wrongly (i.e. not following the guidelines below), resulting in a baby spending every waking moment with a dummy in his mouth and then still using one as toddler, when he should be speaking, not sucking.

When Susan, my first baby, was born and was very unsettled in between feeds, I remember being absolutely amazed when my mother suggested I used a dummy. I couldn't believe that she wanted to see her granddaughter lying around with a dummy in her mouth, so it was with some reservations that I tried using one. I was secretly relieved when Susan immediately spat out the dummy as I felt this showed that she didn't like it and therefore using a dummy was not going to be an option open to me. However, my mother took over and put the dummy straight back into Susan's mouth and, within minutes, my crying, unsettled baby was sound asleep. I was converted!

Some babies are very 'sucky', and find it hard to settle and stay asleep unless they have something to suck on. If your baby is very unsettled (but not hungry) you will find it is far nicer for everyone (including him) to lie him peacefully in his Moses basket with a dummy, rather than having him permanently latched on to your breast, using you as his dummy.

This, therefore, is my recommendation: if your baby needs that extra comfort of a dummy, use one. If he doesn't, don't.

When it comes to using dummies there are several important rules you should follow:

- You should not use a dummy to settle a baby who is due a feed or who is still hungry at the end of a feed. This baby needs food and to deprive him of this is against all the principles of 'demand feeding' and may result in your milk supply diminishing due to lack of stimulation.
- Only use a dummy if you cannot settle your baby without one. Don't automatically put it in his mouth every time you lie him down to sleep – wait and see if he can settle without it.
- Only use it to help your baby to sleep when he needs to sleep.
- Do not use it just to stop your baby crying, e.g. when you are changing his nappy.
- You are unlikely to need a dummy (and therefore should not use one) when you are walking your baby in a pram or buggy, as the movement should rock him to sleep.

If you follow these guidelines, your baby is unlikely to become addicted to the dummy and will usually stop using it of his own accord once he no longer needs it. What normally happens is that by the age of about three months, a baby will either stop needing something to suck on before going to sleep, or he will have discovered his thumb and use that instead. But if your baby does not abandon the dummy of his own volition by about three months, I would recommend that you try to wean him off it, as prolonged use may have a detrimental effect on his teeth, development, etc.

Note: Dummies need to be washed and sterilised frequently. Putting the dummy in your own mouth and sucking on it (as so many mothers seem to do) does not make it germ-free and safe to go back in your baby's mouth – this particularly applies if you have a cold or any other infection, which may then be transmitted to your baby.

Recent research also suggests that a common bacterium frequently found in saliva may be a contributory factor to cot death – **it is therefore inadvisable to lick anything before putting it into a baby's mouth**.

Expressing milk

Before having their babies, many mothers happily assume that they will breast-feed most of the time and be able to give bottles of expressed milk whenever it is not convenient to feed.

Unfortunately, this isn't always as easy to do as you might think. Once your baby is born, you will quickly realise that most of your day seems to be taken up with feeding, winding and nappy changing, and there is little time left for expressing. You may also find that, even if you do have the time and energy to contemplate expressing milk, you don't have any spare milk available – this is because many breasts will only produce enough milk for your baby's immediate needs and little or nothing is left at the end of a feed. You can also suffer from the reverse problem of having too much milk, and you may find that expressing has the undesired effect of stimulating your breasts to the point of making you engorged and at risk of developing mastitis.

Luckily, most mothers can in fact combine breast-feeding with expressing, and many find that by doing this they have the best of both worlds – i.e. their baby only receives breast milk but the mother does not have to do all the feeds herself.

Although it is usually best to wait until breast-feeding is well established before you start planning to express, situations may arise (see below) that precipitate matters. For this reason, it is quite a good idea to research the different types of breast pumps available (see page 7) and possibly buy one in advance so that you are prepared.

You might suddenly find that you need a breast pump for any of the following reasons:

- Your baby is unable to latch on and you need to express your milk and give it to him in a bottle.
- Your nipples become so sore that you are temporarily unable to breast-feed.
- Your breasts become very engorged and you need to express some milk before your baby can latch on.

- You have blocked milk ducts (a pump may help to clear them).
- Your baby is too sleepy or tired to empty your breasts fully at every feed and you temporarily need to do the job for him.
- Your milk supply is low (it may improve if you try to express milk after every feed).

Breast milk *can* be expressed by hand, but most mothers find that this takes too long and they prefer to use a pump if they are expressing on a regular basis.

Whichever method you use, the milk you express can be stored in the fridge in a sterile bottle or sterile container for about 48 hours. You can add expressed milk to any milk that you have expressed earlier on in the day, but if you do this, the expiry time for the milk will be 48 hours from the *first* milk you expressed. Any milk not used within 48 hours should be thrown away. Breast milk can also be frozen for about three months in sterile containers or special freezer bags that you can buy from chemists.

Note: Recommendations for the length of time that breast milk can safely be stored in a fridge vary from 24 hours to eight days. Nonetheless, I prefer to err on the side of caution and would not risk using milk after about 48 hours, but would ideally use it within 24 hours.

Expressing by hand

This is a skill which some mothers master more easily than others, but it is relatively easy to do once you know how. If you are finding it difficult, do ask your midwife to show you what to do and help you get started.

First of all you need to stimulate your let-down reflex. You do this by spending about 15 seconds or so stroking your breast very gently, working from the top of your breast down towards your nipple. Then, using your thumb and first finger, gently squeeze the areola well behind your nipple, squeezing and releasing alternately until you see drops of milk appearing on your nipple. Then lean slightly forward and continue squeezing and releasing, allowing the milk to squirt or drip into a sterile container. It often works best if you change breasts every time the milk flow slows down, as this will allow time for the next wave of milk to come down without you wasting time trying to express in between these waves. Carry on doing this until you have expressed enough milk for your needs or until the milk is no longer flowing well and your breasts feel fairly empty.

Note: If your milk flows very slowly, it can help to have a warm bath or to put warm flannels on your breasts; both of these will encourage the milk to flow better.

Expressing by pump

Most breast pumps come with full instructions, showing you how to assemble and use the pump and also how to sterilise it. They don't, however, always mention the importance of stimulating your let-down reflex *before* you start pumping. If you put the pump on your breast without first doing this, you may well find that the milk takes a long time to start flowing and in some cases it may not flow at all – this often happens when a breast is very engorged or the mother is very tense and anxious. When you first start expressing, be careful to build up gradually both the strength of the suction and the length of time that you spend expressing – you can traumatise your nipple if you pump for too long or too vigorously. You should also:

- Sit comfortably (you do not need to lean forwards).
- Make sure your nipple is central in the funnel.
- If the pump comes with a soft plastic insert, experiment to see whether it is more comfortable to use the pump with or without it (this will depend on the size and shape of your breast).
- Hold the funnel close enough to your breast to maintain suction, but not so close that it digs into your breast and squashes your milk ducts.
- Swap breasts whenever your milk slows down – you can keep swapping back and forth until you have enough milk.

What time of day to express

There is no set time of day that is ideal for expressing milk. Each mother needs to discover for herself at which point of the day her milk is usually at its most plentiful and to judge whether it suits her to express milk at this time. However, as a general rule, most mothers find that their milk supply is at its best during the morning and that this tends to be the best time to express surplus milk. It is usually best to express straight after a feed to allow plenty of time for the breasts to fill up again in readiness for the next feed.

Myths and facts associated with expressing

Mothers are given lots of contradictory advice on expressing and it can be hard to know which advice is correct. I have therefore decided it would be helpful to mention some of the most common misconceptions and explain the thinking that lies behind the different views.

1. *You must not express for the first six weeks.*
The reasoning behind this advice seems to be that expressing before the milk supply is fully established will affect the delicate balance of supply and demand and may stimulate the breasts to over-produce. I would agree that this could happen, but only if the mother is expressing excessively and is taking far more milk out of her breasts than her baby is actually drinking. Expressing should not cause a problem if the mother is doing it in order to give the milk to her baby in a bottle – e.g. because he can't latch on, she has sore nipples or she simply wants someone else to give a feed occasionally

2. *You must not express if your breasts are engorged.*
Many mothers suffer from extreme engorgement when their milk first comes in around Day 4 but are usually advised that on no account should they express as this will make the engorgement even worse. This is simply not true – breasts are only stimulated when expressed on a regular basis. In fact, when a mother is in agony from primary engorgement and her baby is unable to empty her breasts, she *should* fully empty both breasts with a breast pump – see Primary engorgement, page 113.

3. *Long-term expressing will reduce your milk supply.*
Again, not strictly true. Many mothers who were not able to breast-feed their baby (perhaps because he was very premature or ill) will report that they *were* able to express for months on end and had no problem with maintaining their supply. But it is equally true that other mothers will say that their milk supply *did* dwindle and that they ended up having to give some formula milk. Of course, the mothers whose milk supply did fail will never know for sure whether expressing was to blame, or whether they would also have struggled to maintain their supply even if they had been fully breast-feeding. For this reason, mothers should not get upset if they find it hard to

keep expressing enough milk, but I would definitely recommend that a mother stops expressing if her supply is failing and she is expressing as a matter of choice rather than necessity.

4. *A baby will* **always** *get more milk out of a breast than a pump will.* Not true! Most good breast pumps are very effective at emptying a breast and will often do a far better job than a sleepy baby. I have regularly expressed milk from a breast at the end of a feed when a baby is still hungry and unsettled, but is either unwilling or unable to carry on sucking for long enough to get the milk he needs – this baby will then happily take the milk from a bottle. However, a *small* proportion of mothers do find it impossible to extract milk with a pump, even though they clearly have plenty of milk and their baby has no problem with breast-feeding. This is thought to be caused by less prolactin being released when expressing (as opposed to breast-feeding), but as this clearly affects some mothers more than others, it is a question of trial and error to see how well expressing works for you.

5. *If you can't express any milk, your breasts must be empty.*
As a general rule I would agree with this statement. If a mother is able to express milk before, after and in between feeds, expressing is clearly not a problem and should provide a fairly accurate indication of how much milk she has and also how fast her milk flows. If this mother then finds that a time comes when she can't express any milk (e.g. at the end of a feed when she thinks she has run out of milk) this would indicate that her breast really is empty. But if a mother has *never* been able to express any milk, she should not assume that this means she has no milk – especially if her baby is happily breast-feeding and gaining weight! Unfortunately, if you are one of these mothers who genuinely can't express, you will, of course, never be able to use a breast pump to determine how much milk you have and you will just have to use your judgement as best you can.

With all the above factors in mind, you can start expressing your milk whenever you want or need to and see how it works for you.

Note: A breast pump allows a mother to see for herself the huge variations in milk flow. Many are surprised to see that their milk squirts out from one or more ducts on the surface of their nipple, while others are dismayed to see that their milk drips out really slowly. Both speeds are totally normal and explains why one mother will be able to feed her baby much more quickly than another.

Introducing a bottle

It is very common for an exclusively breast-fed baby to refuse to take a bottle if he hasn't got used to taking one from a fairly early age, but unfortunately many mothers don't hear about this problem until it happens to them – by which time it's too late! Even if you plan to breast-feed until your baby is old enough to drink from a beaker, there are many reasons why he might need to be given a bottle sooner than this and it will cause a major problem if he is unwilling or unable to take one.

Any of the following could apply:

- Your baby's weight gain is poor and you are advised to offer top-up bottles.
- You don't have enough breast milk and you are unable to increase your supply.
- You are temporarily unable to breast-feed, perhaps because you are ill and/or have to go into hospital.
- You suffer a severe bout of mastitis which temporarily reduces your milk supply.
- You are due to return to work and you will not be able to breast-feed during your working hours.
- You have an important event forthcoming (e.g. a wedding) and you would prefer to be able to leave your baby at home with a carer.

I regularly see mothers who cannot get their baby to take a bottle and it is truly distressful trying to feed a baby who screams every time you put a teat anywhere near his lips. For this reason alone, I would strongly advise all mothers to give their baby a bottle regularly (once breast-feeding is fully established), so that he is just as happy to feed from a bottle as he is to feed from the breast.

To stop your baby rejecting the bottle, you will need to introduce the first bottle within the first three weeks or so of his birth and you should then give the bottle as often as you think is necessary – probably about once every three to four days. At the first hint of your baby rejecting the bottle, you should use it at every feed until he is happily feeding from it again.

I am *not* suggesting that you give your baby formula milk, as this would have a detrimental effect on your breast-feeding. Instead, you should either express enough milk to give the entire feed via a bottle, or you can just express an ounce or two, which you would give at the start of a feed, finishing off with the breast. Although it might seem both time-consuming and annoying to have to give bottles when you're breast-feeding, I can assure you that every minute you spend doing this will be time well spent if it avoids your baby rejecting the bottle at a later date.

Note: Many mothers are told that they must *never* give their breast-fed baby a bottle as this will cause 'nipple–teat confusion' and will ruin breast-feeding. Several studies have now shown that this is not the case and I myself have never come across a baby who was *happily and successfully breast-feeding* and then totally rejected the breast when offered a bottle. It is, however, likely that a baby who is *not* enjoying breast-feeding (owing to latching problems or a poor milk supply) may well start preferring the easier option of the bottle – if your baby shows signs of doing this, then you should, if possible, stop offering him a bottle. This shouldn't cause a problem with bottle rejection at a later date, as these babies will normally happily take to the bottle at any age.

Ideal length of time to breast-feed

The current government recommendation is that a baby should be exclusively breast-fed for six months. However, although it is clearly best to breast-feed for as long as possible, breast-feeding for six months (or more) will not *guarantee* perfect health for your baby. Nonetheless, if you have a very strong family history of allergies I would encourage you to breast-feed for at least six months if you possibly can, and preferably for as long as nine months to a year.

If you can achieve this you will have done very well, but it is important to realise that *any* breast-feeding is better than none – even if you only manage to breast-feed your baby for a week or so, you will still have given him a better start in life than a baby who has received no breast milk at all.

Note: I would point out that the government recommendation of *exclusive* breast-feeding for six months is unrealistic and unachievable for many mothers. Some mothers will find that they are unable to breast-feed for this long (not enough milk, returning to work, etc.)

and many babies will need to start on solids before six months. (See Starting solids, page 180).

Weaning from breast to bottle

There are several different ways to go about making the change from breast-feeding to bottle-feeding and there is no one way that is substantially better than another. This is because there is such a big variation in the way that breasts react to over- or under-stimulation that it's difficult to offer uniform advice that will suit everyone. However, as a general rule you will find that if your milk supply is very abundant you will need to allow plenty of time to wind down breast-feeding gradually. If, on the other hand, you have always struggled to produce enough milk, you will find that your supply will dry up quite quickly as soon as you stop stimulating it with regular feeds.

When deciding how much time to allow for weaning, you will also need to take into account whether you have an absolute deadline by when you must have fully given up breast-feeding (e.g. going back to work). If there is no such deadline you can obviously be a bit more relaxed.

You should allow at least three weeks for weaning if:

● You *do* have a deadline for stopping breast-feeding.
● Your baby has never been given a bottle and might refuse to take one.
● Your milk supply is very plentiful and you become engorged whenever you miss a feed.
● You have had mastitis more than once (if the mastitis was caused by engorgement rather than by incorrect positioning).
● If you are planning to go on holiday without your baby (you won't want the holiday to be spoiled by your breasts leaking milk and feeling over-full and uncomfortable).

Even if none of the above applies to you, it works best to wean your baby gradually over a number of weeks, allowing both of you plenty of time to adjust to the change.

When weaning, you can use any of the following methods:

● You can miss one feed completely and substitute it with a bottle-feed. As soon as you feel that your breasts have adjusted to missing out this feed, you can drop another, making sure that you alternate breast-feeds with bottle-feeds, rather than dropping two breast-feeds in a row. It doesn't matter which feed you drop first, but it usually works best either to drop the feed at which you feel your milk supply is the least good or one that it suits you to miss, e.g. the mid-morning feed.

- You can shorten each feed, so that your breasts are never fully emptied. This will have the effect of making them gradually produce less milk. The less milk your baby takes from the breast at each feed, the more quickly your breasts will reduce production. You will, of course, need to give your baby a top-up bottle at the end of each feed to provide the milk that he is not getting from the breast.

- You can give up breast-feeding overnight simply by stopping feeding altogether and going straight on to full-time bottle-feeding. This is not a method I would recommend, however, because, although it gets it all over very quickly, there is a price to pay. If you choose this method your breasts will almost certainly become extremely engorged and painful and will remain this way for several days until the message eventually filters through to your breasts to stop producing milk. Even when they have got this message, it will still take them a further two or three days to re-absorb the milk. During this time you will feel extremely uncomfortable (to put it mildly!) and you also run the risk of getting mastitis. This is not a good way to stop breast-feeding and is only worth doing if for some reason you don't have time to wind down more gradually. It is also by far the most painful method if you have a plentiful milk supply and have found in the past that you only had to miss one feed before your breasts became uncomfortably full.

Although it is a matter of personal preference as to which of the above methods you choose, I find the method that works best for most mothers is the first, i.e. dropping entire feeds. The length of time that it takes to wean fully from breast to bottle will depend entirely on how quickly you reduce the amount of time that your baby spends at the breast and how quickly your milk supply dries up. Mothers with a poor milk supply may find that this takes a week or less, while mothers with an abundant milk supply could find that it takes at least a week just to drop one feed comfortably.

It's worth bearing in mind that you can speed up the weaning process at any stage by feeding less, or slow it down by feeding more – remember, the more you feed, the more milk your breasts will produce; the less you feed, the less milk they will produce. If you are unlucky and find that you develop mastitis (even when you have been very careful to reduce feeds slowly), I'm afraid there isn't much you can do, other than take antibiotics and grin and bear it!

Possible weaning problems

● Very occasionally a baby will appear not to tolerate the formula milk very well (e.g. by becoming more 'sicky') and if this happens you should consult your doctor. Although it is unlikely that there is anything wrong with your baby, you may find that a different brand of formula will suit him better than the one you have chosen and your doctor can advise you on this. However, it is much more common for a baby to transfer perfectly happily from breast milk to formula milk without suffering any digestive problems.

● If your baby has not been given a bottle regularly from birth he may well be very reluctant to take his feeds from the bottle (see Refusing bottles, page 156). If this happens you will usually find that it is the bottle that your baby is objecting to rather than its contents – you can test this theory by putting expressed breast milk in the bottle to see whether it makes any difference.

● Your baby might take much less milk at each feed than the feeding charts recommend. If this happens, you'll need to compare the way your baby fed at the breast with the way he is now feeding from the bottle. In other words, if your baby fed little and often at the breast you will almost certainly find that he wants to do the same with the bottle. He will therefore not take as much milk in one go as you would expect.

● Your baby may start each bottle-feed well but refuse to take the whole bottle. If he then cries and becomes distressed (having always fed calmly and happily at the breast) you should consult a doctor. He might be allergic to the formula milk (in which case you will need to change formula) or he may be suffering from reflux, which was less apparent when you were breast-feeding.

● Your baby might temporarily become a bit constipated. This is no cause for concern, as he will usually adapt to the formula milk quite quickly and the condition will resolve itself. In the meantime, suggestions for treating your baby's constipation can be found on page 153.

Breast-feeding and the working mother

I am always being asked by mothers who are going back to work whether it will be possible to breast-feed every morning and evening and give bottles the rest of the time. Unfortunately, this is not a question that I can answer because some mothers can manage it and others can't! It will all depend on how your breasts react when you start trying to do it.

You might find any of the following:

- Your breasts are perfectly happy to provide plenty of milk for the first and last feed of the day and still feel comfortable during the day when you are not feeding.
- Your breasts become so engorged during the day that you have to take a breast pump in to work with you so that you can express off some of the excess milk – this can then be given to your baby the following day instead of formula milk. If you do this you will need to keep the expressed milk cool in a fridge or freezer bag.
- You need to express milk regularly throughout the day in order to keep your breasts sufficiently stimulated to provide enough milk for the morning and evening feeds.
- The tiredness and stress caused by trying to combine work with breast-feeding has a detrimental effect on your milk supply and it becomes increasingly difficult to produce enough milk for your baby.

As it is impossible to predict how a mother's breasts will react when she goes back to work, it really is a question of trial and error. However, if you are committed to combining work with breast-feeding and you find your milk supply is dwindling, you will need to go back to basics and remember that breast-feeding works on a supply-and-demand basis. In other words, the way to boost your milk supply is either to feed more often or to express more often – if you can do either of these your milk supply should start improving again. If it does not improve you will have to accept that this is one of the downsides of going back to work and there is not much you can do about it.

7 Common feeding problems for mothers

I do not recommend that this chapter should be read in great detail during the antenatal period. Most of the chapter is really only relevant to a mother who is actually having one of the problems described – reading too much about potential problems is more likely to be off-putting than helpful! Instead, I suggest that you just glance at the different subjects covered so that you will know where to look if you need help after your baby is born.

Inverted nipples

A mother is sometimes diagnosed as having an inverted nipple when it is in fact not really inverted at all – a nipple that looks inverted may still work perfectly well once a baby starts sucking on it. You can test to see whether your nipple is inverted by using your fingers to mimic the action of a baby's mouth sucking on your breast. If you can grip your nipple between your fingers, your nipple is not inverted, but if you find that your nipple disappears into your breast and you have nothing to hold on to, then you do have an inverted nipple.

If you realise before you get pregnant that you have got an inverted nipple, you may be able to pull it into better shape by using a small suction contraption (made by Avent) called a Nipplette. This claims to work by permanently lengthening the milk ducts inside your nipple – short milk ducts are the main reason why nipples become inverted. You simply fix the Nipplette over the nipple and then leave it on for as many hours of the day and night as you can – it's not painful to use but it will be noticeable if worn under close-fitting tops. You can buy a Nipplette from most chemists but you can only use it between pregnancies and for the first three months that you are pregnant – it won't work later on in pregnancy because the suction cap will keep slipping off when your breasts start producing colostrum. If you have two inverted nipples, both of which are still completely inverted when your baby is born, you will not be able to feed your baby directly from the breast because he will genuinely be unable to latch on. This doesn't mean that you will have to abandon all ideas of breast-feeding, because you can still give your baby breast milk by expressing with a pump, or you can try using a nipple shield (see page 109), which helps by making your breast a better shape for your baby to latch on to (see following sections).

Baby can't latch on

Quite a number of mothers have difficulty getting their baby on the breast in the first few days, and some never succeed at all. This is usually as a result of the mother having very large, flat or inverted nipples, which can make life much more difficult for the baby than small, well-shaped nipples. Having said this, it is in fact fairly easy to get a baby on virtually any shape of nipple provided he is given the help he needs. This will involve shaping your nipple to make it easier for your baby to get it in his mouth.

Over the years I have had many tearful phone calls from mothers who are distraught to find that they are not able to get the baby on the breast. The mother will often think that the main reason her baby can't latch on is because he is not opening his mouth wide enough.

Actually, the real issue is that trying to latch a baby on to a large breast with flat nipples without helping him is the equivalent of expecting him to take the first bite out of an apple! However, if you were to squeeze the apple to make it more the shape of a doughnut your baby would find it very easy to get it into his mouth. It therefore follows that if your baby cannot get his mouth around your large nipple, you will need to make it a better shape for him – you can do this very easily with almost all breasts by using your fingers. It involves exactly the same principle as trying to post a slightly too bulky parcel into a letter box – you would squash the parcel, rather than simply giving up because the opening is too narrow!

Shaping the nipple with your fingers

1. Lift your breast and place it on a pillow with your nipple as far into the centre of the pillow as possible (see page 29).

2. Lie your baby on the pillow, with his body close against yours and his mouth (not his nose) one inch away from your nipple (see *Baby lying with mouth directly in front of nipple*, page 29).

3. Shape your nipple, using the hand which is on the same side as the breast your baby is about to feed from.

4. Place your hand underneath your breast and use the balls of your thumb and third finger to shape your breast. To create the right shape (i.e. to match your baby's mouth) your thumb and finger should be level with your nipple and just on the outside of your areola at the 3 o'clock and 9 o'clock position. You do not want to hold your nipple any closer than this otherwise your fingers will be in the way of your baby's mouth (see below).

5. Gently squeeze your areola until your nipple protrudes – if you squeeze too hard, you may make your nipple invert.

Shaping the breast

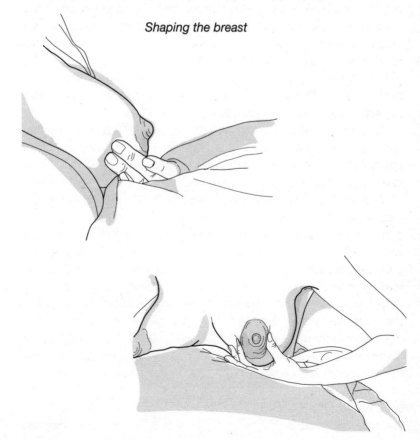

6. Hold your baby's head and shoulders firmly (but not roughly) so that you have good control of his head and can easily direct him towards your nipple.

7. Brush your nipple against your baby's lips and, as soon as he opens his mouth, move him quickly towards your nipple so that you get as much nipple as possible into his mouth before he closes it. I describe this procedure as 'shape and shove'!

8. If your baby closes his mouth on the wrong bit of your nipple, or if he misses it completely, you will need to move him back an inch or two so you can check that you are bringing him straight towards your nipple. Try again but don't be discouraged if it takes several attempts before you both get it right – you are unlikely to get it right first time.

9. Once your baby is on, you can **gradually** let go of your breast and remove your hand – but don't let go too quickly, or he may be pushed off as your breast flattens out again! Once you have removed your hand, you may need to plump up the pillow where it got squashed down by your hand.

If your baby manages to stay on, relax your shoulders and carry on feeding. If he comes off when you let go of your breast, you will need to go back to step one and release your breast more slowly once he starts sucking. If he keeps coming off, check that you have got him lined up so that the nipple is going straight into his mouth and also check that your nipple is level with his mouth. A baby will often lunge upwards as you bring him to the breast (I don't know why), so if he keeps missing, try bringing him to the breast from below the nipple. If you still can't get him on, try asking your husband to help. Men tend to be very technical and are usually very good at this lining-up business!

The 'nose to nipple' theory
I find it absolutely extraordinary that so many mothers are being told to line up their baby 'nose to nipple' rather than 'mouth to nipple'. This never used to be the way it was done and, in my opinion, this advice is the main reason why so many mothers find it hard to latch their baby on to the breast easily and painlessly. In the past, mothers were told that brushing their nipple against the baby's lips would encourage him to open his mouth and this certainly worked. But nowadays, for reasons that are quite beyond my comprehension,

mothers are told to brush their nipple against the baby's *nose* and then wait until his mouth 'gapes wide open' before allowing him to latch on.

I am totally against this advice for the following reasons:

- Lining your baby up with his nose (rather than his mouth) in front of your nipple makes it much harder for him to latch on
- If he does manage to latch on, he will have to pull your nipple away from his nose towards his mouth and this will quickly make your nipples sore
- Latching on this badly, your milk flow will be impeded and feeds will last longer
- Your breast may empty unevenly and this can cause mastitis
- Many babies don't know that they must open their mouth really wide and these babies become very agitated and upset if they are made to wait until they do. In fact, some babies never open their mouth wide and it is up to you to help them latch on by shaping your breast (see Baby can't latch on, page 102).

Every time I see a client who has been taught this method, it takes a matter of minutes to show her that 'mouth to nipple' works better. I also point out that if she was bottle-feeding her baby, she would never dream of irritating him by flicking the teat against his nose and then refusing to put it in his mouth until she deems that he has opened it wide enough! So why do this to a breast-fed baby?

I have come to the conclusion that this 'nose to nipple' theory has evolved from a misinterpretation of the original advice, which recommended that the baby's nose and top lip should be *in line* with the nipple and that he should be lying with his body turned towards his mother so that he is not having to twist his neck to reach the breast. This commonsense advice has been turned into the catchy phrase 'tummy to mummy/chest to chest/nose to nipple/chin to breast' which is then interpreted as meaning the baby's nose should be directly in front of the nipple, rather than in line with it. This is an entirely different concept and I would advise mothers not to be misled if they receive this advice.

Using a nipple shield
If you can't manage to get your baby on the breast by shaping your nipple with your fingers, your next best option is to try using a nipple

shield (see pages 8 and 109). The shape of the shield (see below) will make it fairly easy for your baby to latch on and the suction he exerts as he sucks will often pull your nipple into a better shape. If this happens, you may find that you can remove the nipple shield after a few minutes and then be able to latch your baby directly on to your breast.

But if you can't get your baby to latch on to your breast, you can still carry on using the nipple shield for the entire feed, providing your milk flows well enough through it for your baby to get the milk as easily as he would when feeding directly from your breast. If your feeds don't last too long and your baby's weight gain is fine, you could even continue using nipple shields for as long as you wish to continue breast-feeding. (See page 109 to judge whether the nipple shield is working well enough for you to use it indefinitely.)

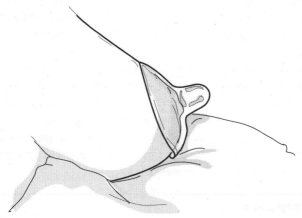

A nipple shield

Expressing

If you can't get your baby on the breast and he is not getting enough milk through the nipple shields, your final option is to try expressing with a pump (see pages 7 and 91). If you do this immediately before a feed, you may find that the pump pulls your nipple out enough to enable your baby to latch on.

Initially, you can try using the pump for only a few minutes, but if this isn't enough to pull your nipple out, increase the length of time you pump. As soon as your nipple becomes a better shape, stop pumping and quickly try to put your baby on the breast while your nipple is still sticking out. The longer you spend using the pump at the start of each feed, the more milk you will be expressing. This doesn't matter too much because any milk you express can be given to your baby at the end of the feed if he is still hungry and your breasts feel empty.

If you find that using a pump at the start of each feed doesn't work, try using it to express the entire feed for several days. This might prove to be more effective in improving your nipple shape – all the milk you express can then be given in a bottle.

If your baby still can't latch on, at some stage you will need to make a decision about what you want to do. If you find it easy to express milk with a pump and are happy to carry on doing this, there is no need for you even to think about giving up breast-feeding and you can be comforted by the fact that your baby is getting the full benefit of your breast milk, albeit via a bottle. But if you find it hard to express enough milk and/or you are becoming increasingly fed up with the amount of time you are spending fiddling around with breast pumps, sterilising bottles and doing feeds, it might be a good decision to call it a day.

If you do decide to stop breast-feeding, you don't have to do it overnight – it normally works better if you gradually reduce the length and frequency of expressing, so that your breasts gradually reduce the amount of milk they are producing and don't become engorged. During this weaning period it is perfectly all right to alternate with breast milk and formula milk and you can even give them both at the same feed if necessary.

Sore nipples

If you ask any mother who has suffered the toe-curling pain of sore nipples to describe what it was like, she will probably tell you that it was one of the worst experiences of her life! Most mothers quickly forget the pain of labour, the sleepless nights and the endless nappies, but very few forget the agony of sore nipples. Sore nipples are cited as being one of the main reasons that women give up breast-feeding and this is such a shame because mothers should not suffer from this problem – sore nipples are **not** part and parcel of breast-feeding.

If your baby is latched on correctly, you will rarely experience any pain, so if you *are* suffering from sore nipples, you should know that this would almost exclusively be the result of:

- incorrect latching on at the breast
- the excessively long feeds that can result from incorrect positioning
- a mother having exceptionally delicate nipples (this would be most unusual)
- nipples infected with thrush or other skin problems
- white nipple (see page 178).

There are many different degrees of pain involved with sore nipples and it is therefore helpful to distinguish between mild nipple pain and the more severe pain which may ultimately prompt the mother to give up breast-feeding.

Types of sore nipples
- The nipples feel a little tender, and feeding is uncomfortable, but bearable.
- The nipples look and feel bruised.
- The nipples are sore, cracked and bleeding, and feeding becomes increasingly unbearable.
- The nipples are tender and pinkish-coloured and there may be shooting pains in the breast during or after feeding. This is more likely to be caused by thrush than incorrect positioning and can be cured by using a suitable fungicidal cream prescribed by your GP.
- From the very first feed, and within only a minute or two of the baby latching on, small clear blisters appear on the end of the nipples. This will normally only happen to a mother who has extremely sensitive and delicate nipples and does not necessarily mean that the baby is latched on incorrectly.
- Your nipple loses colour and turns white, causing extreme pain (see White nipple, page 178).

Note: If your nipples have become so cracked and sore that they bleed during feeds, you may notice your baby possetting up some blood. Swallowing blood is unlikely to cause your baby any harm and it is therefore absolutely fine to carry on breast-feeding as long as you are able to cope with the pain.

Preventing sore nipples
I really cannot stress enough that sore nipples are almost always the

result of incorrect and poor latching of the baby on to the breast. The Royal College of Midwives makes this point over and over again in their handbook – they also point out that the large numbers of mothers who develop sore nipples while still in hospital would suggest that not only are many babies badly attached to the breast but also that many midwives cannot tell the difference between a good and a bad latch. For this reason I would urge any mother who is suffering to keep asking for help and to be aware that once she perfects her technique, the pain should go.

I suggest that you are also aware of the following:

- Unduly long feeds (regularly more than ½ an hour before your milk comes in and longer than one hour after your milk comes in) are likely to be your first indication that your baby may be latched on badly.
- Your nipples should not become sore if your baby latches on correctly.
- Primary engorgement and/or mastitis are often the result of poor latching.
- Using a nipple cream (see page 6) may aid healing, but ultimately correct attachment of the baby to the breast is the essential factor.

Coping with sore nipples

Nipples that are not too badly damaged will usually toughen up over time, even if you continue to do all the feeds and even if your feeding technique remains slightly wrong. But agonisingly sore nipples may need to be given several days' respite to allow them to recover enough for you to continue feeding – they *will* heal (usually within about 24 to 48 hours) if you stop using them for a few days. Unfortunately, this is not a viable option when you have a baby that needs feeding and breasts that are filling up with milk and need regular emptying. What you can do, however, is see whether it is less painful (and therefore less damaging to your nipples) to do a few feeds using nipple shields, or to express milk and give it in a bottle.

Using a nipple shield

It is worth trying nipple shields (see page 8) before you resort to expressing, as they have the advantage (if they work for you) of giving some protection to your nipples while still allowing your baby to feed from the breast, albeit indirectly. This is much more convenient and less time-consuming than expressing and then giving the expressed milk in a bottle.

Some hospitals are reluctant to suggest using nipple shields on the basis that they might affect the baby's sucking reflex and will sometimes reduce the milk supply – some health professionals go even further and say that they should *never* be used. This is most unfortunate, as nipple shields frequently work extremely well and many mothers will recount how they were the miracle answer and enabled them to carry on breast-feeding when they would otherwise have given up.

The success or failure of using shields will depend almost entirely on the mother's let-down reflex – if she is lucky enough to have a fast let-down (which means the milk flows very quickly) her baby will have no problem feeding through a shield. But if her milk flow is very slow, he *will* find it hard to get as much milk out through a nipple shield as he would get if he were feeding directly from the breast, in which case I would be the first to agree that it would be unwise to continue using a shield. I have not, however, found that nipple shields affect the way a baby subsequently sucks at the breast, and feel that they are always worth trying.

Most chemists sell nipple shields and some hospitals do still keep them on the ward and will show you how to use them if you ask. Ideally, they should be sterilised every time they are used but this is not essential – washing them immediately before use with hot soapy water and then drying them with a clean paper towel should be perfectly safe.

The way to tell whether your milk is flowing adequately through the shield is to allow your baby to suck for several minutes and then take him off so you can see whether there is any milk visible inside the shield.

- If there is a pool of milk in the shield, your baby is almost certainly getting the milk easily and you should be able to do the whole feed using it.
- If no milk at all is visible in the shield, you should stop using it immediately – there is no point using it when it is obvious that your baby can't get any milk through it.
- If you can only see traces of milk, your feeds start lasting a lot longer than usual and/or your baby appears more unsettled, this

is a pretty good indication that he is not getting enough milk through the nipple shield and you should stop using it.

- Ultimately, your best guide as to success or failure when using nipple shields is to see how long your baby feeds and how well he settles after a feed – the quicker he feeds and the longer he lasts in between feeds, the better the shields are working.

Ideally, you would only need to use a nipple shield for a few feeds before your nipples heal up enough for you to dispense with it. Often using a shield in this way can get you through what is only a temporary problem and you can then carry on feeding without any further soreness. However, if the reason you got sore in the first place was because your positioning was extremely incorrect, you are likely to get sore again as soon as you stop using nipple shields. If this happens, you will need to go back to basics and continue to try to improve your feeding position (see page 24).

Note: Nipple shields should never be used before the milk comes in as your baby will be unable to get colostrum through a shield.

Expressing with a breast pump

If nipple shields don't work for you, the next thing to try is a breast pump (see page 91) – a breast pump will normally cause less damage to your breasts than a badly positioned baby and will still allow you to feed your baby with your own breast milk.

Once your nipples have recovered, you can try putting your baby back to the breast for some or all of your feeds to see whether you are able to continue without getting sore again. If you do get sore again, you will need to carry on using the breast pump a bit longer before trying again.

Expressing by hand

If you find it too painful to use a breast pump, even with the suction on its lowest level, expressing by hand might be your only option (see page 90).

Using nipple shields or a breast pump for a few days will allow most mothers to recover from sore nipples. If, however, your nipples get sore every time you resume breast-feeding, you will need to think about how much longer you are prepared to carry on in this way. Some mothers are willing and able to go on for many months using a shield or breast pump but others find it too time-consuming and traumatic, and make the decision to stop. It is really down to each individual to decide how well she is coping, but if you do give up breast-feeding, you should try not to feel either guilty or a failure. Instead, it would be more sensible to realise that if no health professional has been able to show you how to latch your baby on painlessly, it is hardly surprising that you gave up on such a miserable experience.

Case History 5
Jessica Cook and Jack (aged 3 weeks)

Jack was Jessica's fourth baby and, as Jessica had had no problems at all with breast-feeding her first three babies, she had no reason to anticipate any problems with this one. Unfortunately, right from the word go, she developed sore nipples. As the days went by, her nipples became so sore, cracked and bleeding that every feed became a nightmare. She was on the point of giving up breast-feeding when a friend recommended that she should consult me.

When I visited her the following day, Jessica was in such agony that she was afraid to put her baby anywhere near her breast. Nonetheless, she reluctantly allowed me to put Jack on the breast and was amazed to discover that, after the initial shock of the first few sucks, the rest of the feed was completely pain-free. It took a couple more visits before she was able to get Jack latched on correctly at every feed but, once she did, her sore nipples healed within a couple of days and she was able to carry on breast-feeding for many months.

Jessica couldn't understand how she could have got her feeding technique wrong with her fourth baby, having got it right with the first three. I pointed out to her that she had aged quite a bit between having her first and fourth baby and that her breasts had no doubt succumbed to gravity and were no longer the same shape and size as they once had been! This meant that she now needed to hold Jack at a slightly different height and angle than had been appropriate for her previous three babies.

Conclusion: *Incorrect positioning causes sore nipples and it is not only first-time mothers who find it hard to get it right.*

Primary engorgement

This is a condition where the breasts get over-full with milk and become extremely hard and painful as a result. If you are unlucky enough to suffer from engorgement, you will find that it occurs when your milk first comes in (usually around Day 3 or 4) and your breasts are filling up with milk faster than your baby is emptying them. This may well happen if your milk comes in very quickly (you have no control over this), and/or when your breasts start off by producing far more milk than your baby needs.

But it is even more likely to occur if your baby is latching on incorrectly and is therefore not emptying the breasts effectively – if you have sore nipples, I'm afraid you will probably get engorged breasts as well. You can also become engorged if you are missing out some breast feeds, e.g. if your baby is being given a bottle at night so you can catch up on sleep.

Prevention

- Ensure that your baby latches on correctly.
- Feed 'on demand' rather than impose a strict four-hourly routine.
- Don't restrict the length of feeds, but do be aware that long feeds (regularly lasting more than one hour) would indicate that your baby is latched on badly and is therefore unlikely to be emptying the breast efficiently.
- Do not miss night feeds as Day 4 approaches.
- If your baby has been unable to latch on and is being fed with formula milk, do make sure that you start expressing your milk as soon as it starts coming in. This will prevent engorgement as well as providing him with your own milk.

If you follow the above advice, you are unlikely to suffer engorgement. Unfortunately, many mothers become engorged before they realise that this is a possible complication of breast-feeding, in which case the next step is to know what to do if you *do* become engorged.

The ultimate cure for engorged breasts is for your baby to empty them, but sometimes this can be easier said than done if he is latched on badly and you are too sore to feed, or if he is having problems latching on at all because your breasts are so over-full with milk that the nipple becomes flattened.

Treatment

● If your baby can't latch on, you could try using a nipple shield. This will provide something for your baby to latch on to and, if your milk flow is good, it should allow him to get the milk as easily as he would when feeding directly from the breast. Ideally you would only use the shield at the start of the feed and then, once your breast has emptied a bit and softened up, your baby should find it easier to latch on – you can then dispense with the shield for the remainder of the feed.

● If your baby *can't* get the milk through the nipple shield, your next best option is to express a bit of milk (by hand or with a pump) before putting him on the breast. This will help to soften the area behind your nipple and make it easier for him to latch on. It will also encourage your milk to start flowing, enabling your baby to get milk easily as soon as he starts sucking.

● If your breasts still feel just as hard and uncomfortable at the end of the feed as they did at the start, this would indicate that your baby is not emptying your breast properly. This theory would be born out if your baby still appears hungry and unsettled even after a really long feed. If this happens, you should express your milk with a pump and offer it to your baby in a bottle – if he *is* still hungry he will drink it and then go to sleep. You will need to keep doing this until your baby manages to empty the breast himself.

● If your baby is breast-feeding well but your breasts still feel fairly full (but not rock hard and solid) at the end of the feed, it is best not to express off the excess milk. Expressing milk after every feed will stimulate your breasts to produce even more milk and you will make the engorgement worse, not better. If you leave your breasts alone they will normally regulate themselves and settle down after a few days.

● If you are very uncomfortable you can take a mild painkiller such as paracetamol. You can also put cold cabbage leaves or special gel pads (available from chemists) into your bra – this will not resolve the problem but will help reduce inflammation and make you feel a bit better.

● A good supporting bra with wide shoulder straps is essential.

With the correct management (as above) primary engorgement usually causes minimal pain and discomfort and will only be an issue for 24 to 48 hours, whereas severe engorgement managed incorrectly can cause real problems. Unfortunately, many mothers are given the wrong advice, namely that on no account must they express as this will only make the engorgement worse. **This is simply not true! Expressing to relieve severe engorgement does *not* stimulate the milk supply.**

If, however, a breast is allowed to become severely engorged, the following can happen:

- The milk sacs in the breasts can become so full that they are unable to contract and expel the milk down into the milk ducts. When this happens, neither your baby nor a breast pump will be able to empty the breast.
- The breasts then become agonisingly painful and there is nothing that can be done to resolve the situation. Nature has to be left to run its course and it usually takes several days before the breasts soften up and the pain subsides.
- As little or no breast milk is obtainable during this time, the baby may need to be given some formula milk.
- Engorgement this severe will often trigger off mastitis, requiring a course of antibiotics.
- During this time, lactation is often suppressed. The mother may then face an uphill battle to build up her milk supply once the engorgement subsides.

To prevent all this happening, it is absolutely essential *not* to allow your breasts to become rock hard with engorgement but instead to start expressing sooner rather than later. You should find that all you need to do is empty your breasts fully (i.e. until they are soft and comfortable) once or twice, and by taking off all this excess milk, the problem is usually resolved instantly. If, however, your breasts continue to fill up as fast as you empty them, you should not keep expressing (as this *will* stimulate your supply) but instead you should leave them alone to regulate themselves. If you then develop mastitis, you will have to regard this as unavoidable and treat accordingly.

Case History 6
Juliet Healey and Katie (aged three days)

Juliet rang me in tears almost as soon as she got home from hospital. Katie had been unsettled from birth and had been breast-feeding endlessly. Juliet had sore nipples and her breasts were engorged and painful but she had been told not to express. When I arrived at the house, Katie was screaming with hunger but was now unable to latch on to the breast at all, and Juliet had no breast pump and was in agony. Everyone was distraught. It was fortunate that Juliet called me when she did because her breasts were still in working order and I was able to empty her first breast in about 10 minutes, using my own small electric breast pump. We then expressed enough milk off her second breast for it to soften up and enable Katie to latch on, and she fed happily (and painlessly!) until she had emptied it completely. We then offered her some of the expressed milk and she was soon asleep.

When I spoke to Juliet the next day she told me that Katie had slept soundly for nearly four hours after I left and had been feeding and sleeping well ever since. Juliet's nipples were already healing up and her breasts were no longer engorged.

Conclusion: *Fully emptying both of Juliet's breasts using a breast pump (and her baby) resolved the problem of engorgement immediately; her breasts did not become engorged again and her milk supply remained good. Giving Katie a bottle of expressed milk when she was only four days old did not cause 'nipple–teat confusion' and affect her ability to suck from the breast. Katie is now four months old and Juliet plans to continue breast-feeding for several more months.*

Case History 7
Sarah Jackson and Harry (aged three days)

Breast-feeding was going well and Harry was happy and settled after each feed. Then it all went wrong. Sarah's milk came in really suddenly on Day 3 and her breasts went from being soft to rock hard within the space of about three hours. Harry could no longer latch on the breast and neither Sarah nor her maternity nurse could express any milk from her breasts, even though they had a top-of-the-range double breast pump.

It was late evening before I was able to visit her, by which time Harry had been given some formula milk to settle him. Sarah's breasts were so hard and her nipples were so flat that there was no way Harry could latch on and, as no milk was flowing at all, nipple shields were not an option. I, too, found that the pump was not able to extract any milk so I had to express by hand, gently pushing back the swollen area around the nipple in order to get my fingers in the right place. Eventually the milk started flowing and the pump was able to take over – we expressed 300 ml (10 oz) of milk from one breast!

Unfortunately, we did not have the same success with the second breast and were only able to express about 30 ml (1 oz). There was nothing else we could do, which meant that Sarah spent the rest of the night in extreme discomfort and by the following morning she had developed mastitis in that breast.

It took a course of antibiotics and at least three days for the pain and inflammation to subside, during which time Sarah continued to find it hard to express any milk from that breast and Harry got very upset whenever she tried to feed him from that side. Luckily, the unaffected breast was working perfectly and Harry was able to get enough milk from that breast to avoid the need for any more formula. It took another two weeks before Sarah's breast recovered and, once the milk started flowing better, Harry was happy to feed from it.

Conclusion: *When milk comes in this suddenly and in such vast quantities, engorgement is almost inevitable. If, however, Sarah had tried to express her breasts earlier than she did, it is likely (but by no means certain) that she would have been able to empty both breasts relatively easily and the whole episode might have been avoided. It was interesting to observe that the breast we did catch in time and empty fully with the breast pump suffered no further engorgement.*

Vascular engorgement

This affects a small number of mothers and is harder to deal with than straightforward primary engorgement. This is because the breasts, in addition to being swollen with milk, are also congested with an increased blood supply and oedema (fluid in the tissues).

The result of this congestion is that milk ducts can become compressed, reducing the milk flow and, in some extreme cases, stopping it altogether. If this happens, you may find that neither your baby nor a breast pump will be able to remove the milk and you may develop some or all of the problems associated with primary engorgement (see page 115).

It is important to make continued efforts to empty your breasts regularly, but if you cannot supply your baby with enough milk you may need to give him some formula milk from a bottle as a temporary measure until the engorgement subsides. Vascular engorgement usually resolves itself within 24 to 48 hours.

Pain relief for vascular engorgement is the same as for primary engorgement, i.e. paracetamol, cold cabbage leaves/gel pads and a good supporting bra.

Note: Even in severe cases of vascular engorgement, it is usually possible to get some milk out of the breast by expressing by hand (see page 90) – this will often succeed where a pump has failed. If you do try hand expressing, be gentle! It is very important not to traumatise further an engorged breast by handling it roughly as this will only make matters worse.

Blocked milk ducts

If you notice very small lumps in your breast (about the size of peppercorns) this would indicate that some of your milk ducts are blocked and are not being emptied properly. These small lumps are usually caused by local inflammation rather than a physical obstruction but the cause and effect are still the same. Initially this will cause no problems but, if left untreated, blocked milk ducts can develop into mastitis.

Milk ducts can become blocked if:

● Your breast becomes very engorged.
● Your baby is latched on badly, resulting in part of your breast not being emptied efficiently.
● You miss a feed (e.g. during the night) so your breast goes too long without being emptied.
● Your bra is too tight or has seams that are digging into your breast.
● You are pressing your breast with a finger throughout each feed to stop your breast smothering your baby's nose – this compresses the milk ducts and prevents that section of the breast from being emptied.

Things to try

● Check that your baby is latching on correctly and/or change the angle at which you are feeding him, e.g. you could try the football hold for a couple of feeds.

● As your baby sucks, gently massage your breast over the lumps and down towards your nipple, using your fingers or a wide-toothed comb.

● Try to empty the breast fully with an electric breast pump. This will usually empty your breast more completely and more evenly than a baby who is latched on badly.

● Change to a bigger and/or seamless bra.

● Don't press on your breast while you are feeding.

If you cannot clear the ducts within one or two feeds, you should consult your midwife, health visitor or feeding counsellor. If the lumpy area remains, becomes red and hot to the touch and you develop a temperature, consult your GP immediately – you may be developing infective mastitis in which case you will need to start on a course of antibiotics. You should still carry on breast-feeding, as the best way to cure blocked ducts is efficient and regular emptying of the breasts.

Mastitis

This is an inflammation of the breast, which can, if left untreated, become infected and even develop into an abscess. If recognised early enough and managed correctly, a mild bout of mastitis may cause few problems and be resolved quite quickly. But severe mastitis can make a mother feel extremely unwell, reduce her milk supply and require a course of antibiotics. Mastitis is almost always caused by the breast not being emptied properly either as a result of severe engorgement and/or by poor attachment of the baby to the breast. In fact, anything that prevents proper emptying of the breast can trigger off a bout of mastitis. In addition, sore nipples can make breasts more vulnerable to mastitis by allowing bacteria to enter through the damaged skin.

Occasionally a mother will develop mastitis for no obvious reason, in which case she has to put it down to bad luck and hope it won't happen again.

The first signs of mastitis developing are blocked milk ducts (see above) or the appearance of a red patch or red streaks on the breast.

This may feel hot and painful to the touch and be accompanied by aching, flu-like symptoms and a high temperature.

Because mastitis is mainly caused by too much milk accumulating in the breast, it is absolutely vital to empty the breast as quickly and as efficiently as possible – by doing this you may well be able to avoid taking antibiotics. If you are able to empty the breast and your symptoms subside, no further action needs to be taken.

But if your symptoms do not improve within 12 to 24 hours you should see your GP as soon as possible as you will need antibiotics, and the sooner you start taking them, the sooner the infection will clear up. If you avoid taking antibiotics you are running the risk of going on to develop an abscess. Not only is it perfectly safe to carry on breast-feeding while you are taking antibiotics but it is far better to do so as this will prevent your breasts from becoming further inflamed. It should take about 24 hours for your temperature to go down and for you to start feeling better, but if there is little or no improvement after two to three days, you should see your GP again as you may need a different type of antibiotic.

If mastitis is caught early enough (and you are given the right antibiotics) you should find that, apart from feeling unwell for 24 hours or so, you will be able to carry on breast-feeding without any undue problems. But if you suffer a severe bout you may find that the affected breast remains very hard and painful for several days and your baby may also refuse to feed from that side – usually out of frustration because the milk is not flowing well. If this happens, you should try to empty the breast at each feed time (either by hand or using a breast pump), but don't be discouraged if you find it hard to express much milk from your breast. It is very common for this to happen and you may find that it takes a week or more for your milk flow to improve again and for your supply to return to normal. During this time your baby may be able to get enough milk for his needs from your unaffected breast but if he can't, you will need to supplement his feeds with some formula milk until your supply improves.

If you are feeling very unwell, do be kind to yourself! It is a good idea to go to bed for a few days, taking your baby with you and feeding him more frequently – but don't feed your baby in bed if you're at risk of falling asleep. You should also increase your fluid intake, and putting warm compresses on your breast will both relieve the pain and improve the milk flow. Ibuprofen is probably the best analgesic to use as this will help reduce inflammation as well as providing pain relief.

Getting mastitis once is usually just bad luck, but if it follows on from sore nipples and/or you get mastitis more than once, it may be that you are not getting your feeding position right. Keep trying to correct your positioning (see page 24) because if you don't, you are likely to get recurrent mastitis and this will have a very detrimental effect both on your morale and your ability to sustain breast-feeding.

However, some mothers, through no fault of their own, are extremely prone to mastitis and there is nothing that can be done about this other than treating each infection with antibiotics. If you do get recurrent attacks it's worth consulting a specialist (your GP should be able to refer you to one), but don't expect miracles! In my experience, even a specialist cannot always find a solution for vulnerable breasts and I know of several mothers who have ultimately been advised to stop breast-feeding rather than continue to take antibiotics on such a regular basis.

Note: A small amount of the antibiotics will pass through into the breast milk and this might give your baby diarrhoea and will also make him temporarily more susceptible to thrush. Although these side effects are, of course, undesirable, they will do your baby no harm and it is better to continue breast-feeding than to introduce formula milk at this point. See Drugs and Breast-feeding, page 74.

Breast abscess

If mastitis is not treated with antibiotics, an abscess can form, either just below the surface near the areola, or deeper down within the breast tissue. If this happens, you will need to go into hospital to have it incised and drained, usually under a general anaesthetic. Provided the incision is not too close to the nipple, you should be able to continue breast-feeding and if you can, this is likely to speed up the healing process. If you find it too painful to breast-feed, you should express the milk by hand or pump from the affected side, while still continuing to feed from the unaffected breast.

Note: You should always confirm with your consultant that it is all right for you to continue to breast-feed and also that it is safe for your baby to have the breast milk from the affected side. This is because in some cases he may feel that the milk has been contaminated and that it's better to wait a day or two before your baby starts having the milk. If you have to throw away all the milk that you express, you will need to give your baby some formula to supplement your feeds until you are fully breast-feeding again.

Too much milk

If you find that your breasts are producing so much milk that they constantly feel over-full and uncomfortable and leak a lot in between feeds, you will want to know what can be done about it. You are unlikely to get much sympathy from other nursing mothers, as they will probably feel envious! This is a bit tough, because having too much milk can be just as big a problem as having too little, even if it doesn't appear so to anyone else.

Unfortunately, there is nothing much that you can do to stop your breasts from over-producing, other than to wait for them to regulate themselves. It will normally take two to three days for your breasts to get the message that they are producing much more milk than your baby needs and to slow down production. A small number of mothers may experience several weeks of discomfort before their breasts adjust and start feeling significantly more comfortable.

Things to try

- Wear a good supporting bra.
- Express a small amount of milk in between feeds if you are feeling excessively uncomfortable.
- Try not to express more milk than is absolutely necessary for your comfort, because expressing too often will usually stimulate your breasts to produce even more milk.
- If expressing small amounts doesn't help, you could try using a breast pump to empty the breasts completely after one or two feeds. If this doesn't solve the problem (i.e. your breasts still fill up more quickly than your baby can empty them) you should not keep doing this.
- Use breast shells (see page 8) to collect any milk that leaks out – these will be more effective than breast pads and have the added benefit that you can keep any milk that you collect. If you are going to keep the milk (rather than throw it away), you should sterilise the breast shells and empty them regularly.

Mothers are often advised not to express any milk when they are engorged, on the basis that doing so will encourage the breasts to produce even more milk. In my experience this is not the case. It is certainly true that the more milk you remove from the breasts the more milk they will produce, but it's all a question of balance. Expressing a small amount of milk in between feeds will help enormously in terms of relief from the acute discomfort of engorged breasts and should not result in the breasts becoming over-stimulated. If, however, your breasts do not settle down after a few days of moderate expressing, you should stop all expressing and leave them to sort themselves out.

Milk flow is too fast

If your milk flow is very fast and your baby has no problem in coping with it, you don't need to do anything other than enjoy the fact that your feeds won't take very long.

But if your milk is pouring out faster than your baby can comfortably swallow it, it can make feeds very traumatic for both of you and you will need to do something about it. A good indication that your baby is unable to cope is his coming to the breast, sucking for a very short time (e.g. less than a minute or two) and then pulling away crying and appearing distressed. If he keeps doing this he is almost certainly being frightened by the sheer speed at which the milk is flowing and he will probably get more and more panicky with each subsequent feed. If you don't rectify the problem he may become so frightened of the breast that he may start crying before you can even latch him on and, in some extreme cases, may refuse to suck on the breast at all.

There are many different opinions on how best to slow down the flow of milk and everyone you ask is likely to suggest something different. I have found only one method that really works and that is to use a nipple shield (see page 8). This works by containing the milk inside the shield so that it only comes out when your baby actually sucks, rather than pouring directly into his mouth as it would when he feeds normally. You will usually find that as soon as you start using a shield your baby will be transformed into a calm, relaxed baby who feeds slowly and normally from then on. If your milk flows fast through-out the entire feed you will need to use a shield all the time, but if you find your milk slows down after a few minutes (see Using a nipple shield, page 109) you can take the shield off and finish without it.

Note: Your baby may become more able to cope with a fast flow of milk as he gets older, so it's worth trying to feed him without a nipple shield every now and then to see whether he can manage without it.

Case History 8
Philippa Wendell and Georgina (aged 10 weeks)

Georgina was Philippa's first baby. Right from the start, feeds had been fairly fraught, with Georgina regularly crying before, during and after feeds. Each feed time was a battlefield, with Georgina crying and pulling away from the breast and rarely settling for long in between feeds. Philippa was worried that something was wrong with Georgina and had consulted both her GP and health visitor, both of whom said her baby was fine and that she should stop worrying. However, feeding did not improve and crisis point was reached on a Sunday afternoon when Georgina had been crying all day, but would neither feed nor go to sleep. Her parents were on the point of taking her to Casualty when a friend suggested they should consult me.

I went straight round and was confronted by a fraught mother and a crying baby. I put Georgina on the breast, and could immediately hear her gulping and choking on what was obviously an extremely fast flow of milk. She was clearly panicking as she cried and pulled away from the breast. I produced a nipple shield, put Georgina back on the breast and within minutes she was calmly feeding. Philippa was amazed and said that this was the first feed that she had done since Georgina was born that was both calm and relaxed. Georgina fell asleep after the feed, and when I rang Philippa 24 hours later the crisis was over! She wrote me this letter:

Dear Clare,
A short note to thank you so much for coming to my rescue on Sunday. The nipple shield has made all the difference. Georgina now seems a much more relaxed baby – not surprising because the poor thing isn't bunged up with wind! In turn, it is already making a big difference to my life too – as she now sleeps more I can get on with more things and life seems a little less chaotic. I only wish I had met you before!
    Thank you once again.

Kind regards,
Philippa

Conclusion: *Nipple shields can work well in instances where the mother's milk flow is too fast for her baby to cope.*

Not enough breast milk

A mother will often think that she doesn't have enough milk if her baby is not settling well after feeds and is not gaining enough weight. However, I regularly see mothers whose milk supply is fine but whose babies are incorrectly positioned at the breast and are not feeding efficiently – these babies will then often fall asleep before they have fully emptied the breast. So, before leaping to the conclusion that your milk supply is poor and thereby losing your confidence in your ability to provide enough milk for your baby, you should first check the following:

- Is your baby correctly positioned at the breast with enough nipple in his mouth and is he latched on at the correct angle so that your milk can flow freely?
- Are you using both breasts per feed? (See One breast or two?, page 20)
- Are you tiring your baby out by making him spend too long sucking on the first breast (which may be empty) before swapping him to the second?
- Is he feeding for long enough, or is he dozing mid-feed? If your baby regularly falls asleep during feeds, try keeping him awake and see whether by feeding longer, he then settles better. Feeding him in a slightly cooler room and with fewer clothes on will normally help to keep him awake.
- Try doing your nappy change at the halfway stage instead of at the start of the feed – this will also help to keep him awake.
- Try to make sure your baby is getting plenty of sleep between feeds – if he is not getting enough rest he can become too tired to feed properly.

If none of the above helps and your baby remains unsettled and is still not gaining enough weight, it may well be that your milk supply is low. You can confirm this by trying one of two experiments, either of which should give you a very clear indication of how much milk you are producing in comparison with how much milk your baby needs.

Method one

Give your baby a normal-length breast feed (i.e. feed until you would normally stop) and then straight away offer him extra milk from a bottle, without making any attempt to settle him first. Ideally, you would offer him breast milk that you have expressed earlier on that day (or got out of the freezer) but if you have none available, you will have to give him formula milk.

If your baby is still hungry he will immediately become more alert and will feed hungrily from the bottle until he is full. He should then fall sound asleep and not need feeding again for several hours. If your baby does take any milk at all from the bottle, you should then get the breast pump out as soon as possible to see how much milk you have left in your breasts, compared with how much he has just drunk from the bottle. If you cannot begin to match the amount, this almost certainly means that your milk supply is too low.

Method two

Substitute an entire breast feed with a bottle feed. Offer your baby as much as he will take, partly to see how much milk he wants and partly to compare how well he settles after what you know will have been a full feed. As soon as possible after feeding him, you should then express both breasts to see how much milk you have, compared with the amount of milk he has just drunk. Once again, this should give you a pretty good indication of how your supply compares with his needs.

I am aware that not everyone will agree that expressing gives a reliable indication of milk supply (see Expressing milk, page 89) but I have found this to be the easiest and clearest way to identify how much milk a mother has and to see what is going on. I would therefore recommend that a mother tries either of the above methods and makes her own judgement as to how effective it is.

If your milk supply is low you can usually (but not always) improve it by devoting time and energy to the problem. It normally takes at least 24 hours, if not two or three days, for your milk supply to increase, so don't become discouraged if things don't improve overnight.

Things to try

● Make sure you are eating and drinking plenty, and also that you are getting enough rest. Although it is hard to rest if your baby is constantly crying and feeding, you can at least make sure that you are not rushing around doing unnecessary things when you could be resting. Accept that your house may be less tidy than usual and try to get someone else to help with the cooking.

- If possible, retire to bed for a day or two, taking your baby with you. This way, you can concentrate solely on feeding him and keep your energy for making milk.

- You need to give your breasts the message that your baby needs more milk than they are producing. You can do this by feeding longer (but not much longer than an hour) and more frequently, possibly feeding as often as every two hours. Be prepared for it to take a minimum of 24 hours before your breasts respond.

- Allow your baby to continue sucking at the end of each feed, even if your breasts feel empty – this is the best way to give them the message that they should not be empty and that your baby needs more milk. You may need to feed for at least an hour before your baby eventually dozes off to sleep.

- Only offer top-up bottles if you simply cannot settle your baby without one.

All of the above is fairly standard advice that you will get from most health professionals and should be the first things you try. However, in practice you may find some of it hard to implement. This is because the basic premise of stimulating your breasts by feeding longer and more frequently will only work if your baby is willing to play ball! The reality is that many babies are not prepared to keep on sucking on an empty breast – they will either get angry and frustrated once the breast is empty or else they fall asleep because your breast has become a dummy rather than a source of food.

If this happens, I recommend that you use a breast pump as your main tool to stimulate your breasts and improve your supply. This is what you do:

- Allow your baby to suck on the first breast for as long as he continues to suck properly – this can be anything from 5 minutes to 30 minutes, depending on how much milk you have.

- Your baby will usually stop sucking properly (see page 34) when your milk has run out, so this is the time to swap breasts.

- When he stops sucking properly on the second breast, you should try to settle him to sleep.

- If he is still too hungry to settle, you should offer him a top-up bottle.

● You then need to use a breast pump at the end of every feed to express any milk that might be left and to stimulate milk production – any milk you express can be given as a top-up (if needed) at a subsequent feed.

You will notice if your breasts are responding to this stimulation because you will either start expressing more milk or, better still, your baby will gradually reduce the amount of milk he is taking as a top-up. As soon as you reach the point where he no longer requires a top-up, you can stop expressing and resume full breast-feeding, safe in the knowledge that you now have plenty of milk for him.

Unfortunately, things don't always work out this well for everyone and a small proportion of mothers may find that they simply cannot get their breasts to produce enough milk, however hard they try.

If after at least three days there is **absolutely no improvement at all** in your milk supply, I have to say that in my experience it is unlikely that things will get any better. If it becomes obvious that expressing is having no positive effect on your supply, there is little point in continuing to do it. Instead, you should carry on breast-feeding, stop expressing, and top your baby up with formula milk as and when he needs it. You can continue to do this for as many weeks or months as you wish.

Note: The general consensus is that every mother will be able to produce enough milk for her baby, and mothers are therefore made to feel such a failure if they find they can't. I am so saddened by this attitude because I firmly believe that some breasts work much better than others and everything I see on a daily basis continues to support this belief. I regularly visit mothers who start off with so much milk that they could feed several babies and then I see other mothers who have *never* had enough milk – no hint of engorgement and little evidence even to show that their milk has come in at all. I once visited a mother with a four-day-old baby, who was in complete agony with engorged breasts – using a breast pump, I expressed 20 oz (600 ml) of milk in the space of about 20 minutes! Given the fact that a four-day-old baby would normally only need one or two ounces of milk, it would be a complete understatement to point out that these breasts were *hugely* over-producing. It therefore seems logical to me that breasts can go to the other extreme and hugely under-produce. So, please, don't feel you have failed if your breasts let you down. Our bodies are *not* perfect.

Medications that may enhance lactation

There are numerous homeopathic and over-the-counter remedies that claim to boost milk production and are certainly worth trying if all else fails. The feedback that I get from my clients would suggest that in some cases they do seem to be of some help and in other cases the mother notices little or no improvement. You can try drinking four to five cups of fennel tea a day and/or take three fenugreek tablets three times a day – these remedies can be found in good health food shops and some pharmacies. It is best to consult a homeopath if you wish to try a homeopathic preparation as he will be able to advise you as to which remedy is best suited to you.

As a last resort, you could ask your doctor to prescribe Domperidone, which is a drug normally prescibed to treat the nausea and vomiting that are caused by gastrointestinal disorders, but which has also been found to increase milk production in breast-feeding mothers. The recommended dose of domperidone is 10 mg three to four times a day, and it may take up to two weeks for your breasts to respond.

Growth spurts

It is one of the miracles of nature that, when breast-feeding, your breasts will remain pretty much the same size regardless of how much milk they are making and storing – your breasts do not become bigger and bigger as the weeks go by. Breast-milk production, therefore, usually increases gradually to meet your growing baby's needs without you even being aware that this is happening.

However, it is normal for a baby to have the occasional growth spurt when he will suddenly need a lot more milk and, if this happens, your breasts will be put under immediate and unexpected pressure to increase milk production in a very short space of time. These growth spurts usually occur at approximately three weeks, six weeks, three months and six months. If you think that your baby is having a growth spurt, you should increase your food and fluid intake, feed him more frequently and rest more until your milk supply meets the new demands – this will probably take 24 to 48 hours.

Baby 'fussing' at the breast

Breast-feeding should be a peaceful and happy experience. When a mother settles down to feed her baby she expects him to latch on easily and then feed calmly until he is full. Unfortunately, it doesn't always work out like this and it's not that unusual for a mother to find that her baby 'fusses' at the breast – and the more he does this, the more stressful feed times can become. The reasons are numerous:

1. Right from the outset, you find it hard to latch your baby on to the breast. You find that your baby starts crying as soon as you lie him near your breast, his head wobbles around while he frantically tries to latch on to the nipple, but he fails to do so. You may also find that the more you push your baby towards the breast, the more he cries and pulls away. The most likely cause of this behaviour is that you are bringing your baby towards the breast at the wrong angle and/or not shaping your nipple. This makes it hard for him to latch on and it is very frustrating for him. The hungrier he is, the more upset he will get (see Baby can't latch on, page 102).

2. Your baby latches on to the breast fairly well, or even very well, but almost immediately starts crying and pulling away. This tends to happen when your milk is flowing much too fast for your baby (see page 123).

3. Your baby feeds well but then starts crying and pulling off the breast towards the end of the feed, even when you are pretty sure he is still hungry. The most likely cause of this is either that your milk is flowing too slowly, or your breast is empty and you don't have enough milk for him (see page 125).

4. Your baby feeds well but cries and pulls off the breast frequently throughout the feed and appears to be in pain. The most likely reason for this happening is discomfort caused by wind (see page 35), colic (see page 144) or reflux (see page 148).

5. Your baby has breast-fed perfectly well and happily for weeks or even months and then, for no apparent reason, starts crying and fussing at the breast. Typically, he will latch on well but at some point will cry and arch his back and pull away from your breast, often dragging your nipple in his mouth. This is both painful and distressing for you. Sometimes you will find that he will latch on again almost immediately and at other times you have to spend ages calming him down before he will go back to the breast. This

behaviour may only last for a few feeds and then miraculously stop, or it may go on for days until you reach the point where you contemplate giving up breast-feeding. Unfortunately, I don't know why babies do this. It may be that the mother has eaten something (such as garlic) that is making her breast milk taste unpleasant. It could also be that the mother is suffering from stress or has started taking a lot of exercise, both of which (according to recent research) could affect the taste of her milk. Apart from suggesting that you examine your lifestyle and diet, making any necessary changes, there is little that I can advise other than to 'muddle' through and hope that this behaviour doesn't persist for too long.

Of course, if there is anything else about his behaviour that concerns you, I would recommend that you consult your GP.

Baby can't or won't suck efficiently

Some babies start life appearing to be either unable or unwilling to suck at the breast. Most of these babies simply need skilled help to enable them to latch on easily, and from then on breast-feeding will normally progress smoothly. However, in a small number of cases a baby may be slow to get going on the breast and it may take days or even weeks before breast-feeding can be fully established.

The first step is to diagnose the problem and then see what, if anything, can be done about it. The extent of the problem can range from a baby not being able to latch on at all (see Baby can't latch on, page 102) to a baby who appears to latch on to the breast well but then either falls asleep after a few sucks, or continues to suck but in such a feeble way that he gets little or no milk. The latter problem can be caused by any of the following:

- Your baby is not latched on correctly and is therefore not getting the milk easily.
- Your baby is becoming dehydrated and has no energy to suck.
- He has jaundice which is making him too sleepy to feed.
- He is a very sleepy baby and needs to be fed with fewer clothes on.
- Your nipple is so big and hard that he genuinely can't get enough of it into his small mouth (you will need to express milk to keep the supply going until he is big enough to latch on).

- He was born prematurely and needs time to develop a stronger sucking reflex.
- He has a minor defect in his mouth (e.g. tongue-tie) which is preventing him from being able to suck efficiently – your GP or a paediatrician can check this for you.
- He suffered intracranial trauma at birth (minor damage to his head) which is affecting his sucking reflex. A cranial osteopath may be able to resolve this problem.
- He has an infection that needs diagnosing and treating.
- You have little or no milk and your baby is not prepared to suck on an empty breast.

By referring to the relevant sections in this book you should find that you can resolve most of the above issues. However, I do very occasionally come across a healthy full-term baby who simply will not suck on the breast even though he has no problems latching on and even though the mother has plenty of milk. It is extremely frustrating when this happens and I have yet to find the answer to this problem. These babies will often be very poor and 'lazy' feeders who also feed badly from a bottle, regularly taking up to an hour to finish a feed. If this proves to be the case, I will suggest the mother expresses her milk and carries on bottle-feeding in the hope that her baby will gradually speed up and she can make another attempt to establish breast-feeding.

Case History 9
Rosie Best and Freddie (aged two weeks)

Rosie was never able to get Freddie to feed from her breast. She had no problem at all latching him on but Freddie then just lay with her nipple in his mouth and did nothing! Eventually a midwife cup-fed him with some formula milk as he was clearly hungry, but still no one could get him to suck on the breast. Rosie called me in when Freddie was two weeks old to see if I could help. I was easily able to latch him on and Rosie had such a fast milk flow that her milk was dripping into his mouth – and still he wouldn't suck! He was wide awake and hungry but would neither suck on the breast nor on a nipple shield, even though the shield filled up with milk as soon as we put it on.

Conceding defeat, Rosie expressed her milk for the next few months and sadly never managed to get Freddie to feed from her breast.

Two years later Clemmie was born and breast-fed perfectly, right from the very first feed.

Conclusion: *For no obvious reason, some babies can't or won't breast-feed.*

The ill mother

It is normally safe to continue breast-feeding if you are suffering from a common illness such as a cold or flu, but if you develop a more unusual illness (e.g. food poisoning) you should consult a doctor. If he advises you to stop breast-feeding for a few days, you will need to express your breasts at least four-hourly (and throw the milk away) in order to keep your milk supply going until you can start again. In the meantime, your baby can be fed with formula milk.

Mothers who are HIV- or Hepatitis-positive are advised not to breast-feed at all.

8 Common feeding problems for baby

As with the previous chapter, I feel that it would be counter-productive to read the whole of this one during the antenatal period, as it also concentrates on problems and, with a bit of luck, you will not have to read it at all! Nonetheless, it is still worth flicking through the headings so that you know which problems are covered, in case you experience any of them and find that you need help.

Jaundice

It is very common for a baby to suffer a mild degree of jaundice between Days 3 and 5 and it will usually clear up of its own accord by Day 10. You can tell if your baby is becoming jaundiced because his skin and the whites of his eyes will begin to develop a yellowish tinge. If he becomes jaundiced while you are still in hospital the midwives will almost certainly notice it as quickly as you do and will, if necessary, do a blood test to check the level of jaundice.

Jaundice is caused when there is temporarily too much bilirubin (which has a yellow pigment) in the baby's blood. The more bilirubin there is, the more yellow the baby becomes. If his liver is unable to get rid of the bilirubin quickly enough, the baby may need to have phototherapy to reduce the bilirubin levels. Although this can be worrying to a new mother, it will not cause the baby any pain or discomfort.

Phototherapy involves lying the baby naked in his cot either on a fibre-optic blanket or under overhead ultraviolet lights, both of which help break down the bilirubin. The amount of time he will need to spend under the lights will depend on how long it takes for his jaundice to clear up, but usually it won't be for much longer than 24 hours or so after starting treatment. While your baby is under the lights you may be advised by the midwives or a paediatrician to feed him more often (e.g. three-hourly) and you will probably have to wake him for these feeds. Jaundice usually makes a baby very sleepy.

Even if your baby is only slightly jaundiced it is probably still a good idea to feed him three-hourly during the day until his jaundice fades. This is because even a slightly jaundiced baby may be too sleepy to feed as often as he should, with the result that he may wake for fewer feeds than he actually needs. If you allow him to feed too infrequently, you are likely to find that when he recovers from his jaundice he will suddenly want to feed a lot more to make up for all his missed feeds. You may then find that your breasts are not able to cope with this sudden increase in demand.

A jaundiced baby can be quite hard to wake and will frequently fall sound asleep during feeds, long before he has had enough milk. If this happens, you could try feeding him in a slightly cooler room and/or remove some of his clothing during feeding times. It may also help to do a nappy change at the halfway stage of his feed. Remember, it is in your baby's best interests to have plenty of milk, so you mustn't feel that you are being cruel if you use any of these methods to keep him awake and feeding.

If your baby becomes jaundiced at home:

- Point out to the visiting midwife that he is becoming yellow because she may not notice, especially if he is lying in a dimly lit room.
- Ring your midwife if you know that she is not planning to visit you that day and ask her to come and check your baby.
- Ring your midwife again if you are worried that your baby has become more jaundiced since she last checked him.
- If he becomes very jaundiced, he may need a blood test as this is the only completely accurate way of finding out whether the jaundice needs treating. Your district midwife may have the equipment to do the blood test in your home but if she doesn't, you will need to take your baby to hospital to be tested.
- If his jaundice levels are too high, he will need to be admitted to hospital for phototherapy.

● If he is too sleepy to feed efficiently from the breast, you may need to express your milk and bottle-feed him for a few feeds.

Breast milk jaundice
A very small number of babies will develop breast milk jaundice, thought to be caused by the mother having an enzyme in her milk that temporarily stops the bilirubin being expelled effectively. This jaundice is usually mild and does no harm and the bilirubin levels will gradually return to normal over a period of three to ten weeks. If there is any cause for concern, blood tests can be done to exclude liver or thyroid problems, but in most cases the mother can carry on breast-feeding until the condition resolves itself.

Note: If you stop breast-feeding for a couple of days breast milk jaundice will usually disappear very quickly, but it is not normally necessary to do this.

The sleepy baby
If your baby is very sleepy but wakes regularly for feeds, feeds well and gains the right amount of weight, you are extremely lucky and you should enjoy it while it lasts.

If he is temporarily very sleepy with jaundice you should find that he gradually becomes more wakeful as the jaundice wears off, so this is not a long-term problem. You will, however, need to take active measures during this time (see Jaundice, page 135) to ensure that he gets enough milk for his needs.

But if your baby is too sleepy to feed properly and is showing signs of dehydration (see Dehydration, page 155) or is not gaining weight (see Poor weight gain, page 141), you will need to encourage him to feed a bit more, following the advice given in the relevant sections.

Note: If your baby remains abnormally sleepy, you should consult a doctor – he may have an infection (e.g. of the urinary tract) that requires treatment.

The unsettled baby
An unsettled baby, who is constantly demanding attention, is one of the most tiring, demoralising and upsetting things to contend with in the early days of parenthood. Unfortunately, it is not uncommon for a mother to find it hard to settle her baby in the first few weeks – this is mainly due to inexperience and not really knowing what to do if the baby won't go to sleep after a feed. But as a new mother cannot

expect to become an expert overnight, you should not feel inadequate if this happens to you.

In most cases where a baby is unsettled, the mother will feed her baby until he falls sound asleep, but within a very short time of being settled, he is awake again and crying. Presuming that her baby is still hungry, the mother picks him up and puts him back to the breast. Once again she feeds him, winds him, checks his nappy and settles him back down to sleep. Her baby then wakes, starts crying and the poor mother (not knowing what else to do) puts him back to the breast and starts the whole cycle all over again.

If this cycle of endless feeding and crying lasts for only a small part of the occasional day, you may need to accept that you have a fairly unsettled baby who does require quite a lot of attention at certain times and there is probably little that you can do to improve matters. In this case, all you can do on the occasions when he won't settle is to muddle through, feeding, winding, etc., until he goes to sleep. But if this behaviour carries on for more than 12 hours or so, you need to realise that what you are doing is not working and is not the way to settle your baby. In other words, you need to find a solution that does not involve endlessly 'fiddling' with him.

You may find it helpful to know that in the vast majority of cases where a baby gets into this cycle of non-stop feeding and crying, he is usually either:

- hungry
- in need of winding
- overtired and needing to go to sleep
  or
- suffering from discomfort, e.g. colic, reflux or milk intolerance.

If you find that you are getting into a terrible muddle, and you are spending all day and possibly much of the night 'fiddling' with your baby, with each feed merging into the next, don't struggle on, assuming that this is part and parcel of motherhood. Instead, re-read Chapter 3 on how to feed and settle your baby. You should also refer to the sections on milk intolerance, colic and reflux (pages 141–152), consulting a doctor where necessary.

If none of the above helps, you need to establish precisely why your baby is not settling and you can do this by going through the following checklist:

1. *Exclude hunger by offering your baby extra milk.*
Give your baby a normal length breast-feed (i.e. feed until you would normally stop) and then straight away offer him extra milk from a bottle, without making any attempt to settle him first. Ideally, you would offer your baby breast milk that you have expressed earlier on that day, but if you have no breast milk available you will have to give him formula. If he drinks some milk and then falls sound asleep, you will know that hunger was the reason why he would not settle. If this proves to be the case, you should refer to Not enough breast milk, page 125. If he doesn't want any milk, or only takes a very small amount and still doesn't settle, you will know that he is not hungry and you should therefore not keep putting him back to the breast.

2. *Once you have excluded hunger, try winding your baby thoroughly. (See Winding, page 35.)*
If this doesn't settle him to sleep, you will now have established that he is not hungry and does not need winding, and you should therefore concentrate all your efforts into getting him to sleep. Don't offer him any more milk (from breast or bottle), or make any further attempts to wind him.

3. *Try getting your baby to sleep.*
● Swaddle him, offer him a dummy and rock him to sleep.
● Leave him for a few minutes to see whether he needs to cry himself to sleep (see page 41).
● Take him for a walk in his pram or for a trip in the car, either of which should send him to sleep.
● Settle him to sleep on your lap (see below).

When a baby has become so fraught and overtired that he is completely unable to fall asleep using the first three methods described above, the one sure way to give respite to both you and him is to settle him to sleep on your lap. This method works far better than endlessly pacing the room, swapping your baby from shoulder to shoulder and continually putting him down as soon as he dozes off, only to find he is awake again within minutes. The real key to the success of the 'lap' method is that it tends to send your baby into a deeper and more permanent sleep than any other method and is also far less stressful and tiring for the mother.

The first step is to sit comfortably with someone or something (e.g. the television!) to keep you company so that you don't try to rush things. Place a pillow on your lap and lie your baby on his tummy on the pillow, turning his head gently to one side so that you can, if necessary, put a dummy in his mouth (see below). You should then start patting your baby on his back just above the nappy level, firmly and rhythmically, at a rate of approximately one pat per second. Most babies find this very soothing and comforting and will usually fall asleep quite quickly. Don't be discouraged if he cries a lot for the first few minutes because, if you persist with the rhythmic patting, you will find that his crying will diminish and he'll start to fall asleep.

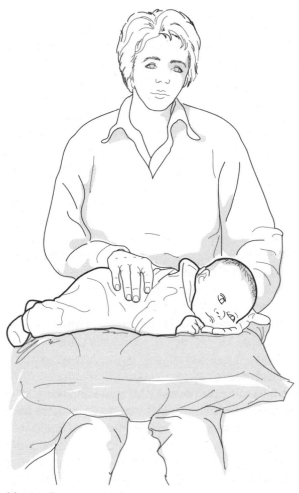

Settling him to sleep on your lap

Once your baby is asleep, you can stop patting him but you should leave him lying on your lap for a few minutes longer to check that he has gone into a sound sleep and has not just dozed off. If he starts stirring and waking, pat him again (but do not pick him up) until he goes back to sleep. If he stays asleep for approximately five minutes after you have stopped patting him, you can pick him up gently and put him into his crib.

If he then remains asleep, you will have achieved your goal and need do nothing further. But if he wakes as soon as he is in his crib, you will need to put him back on your lap and start the process all over again.

If you find that your baby wakes every time you move him to his crib, you may need to leave him sleeping on the pillow until his next feed is due. Ideally, you should be able to move the pillow from your lap and put it (and your baby) on to a surface where he will be safe (e.g. on a sofa, surrounded by cushions) and where he will not be at risk of rolling off. However, an extremely tense and overtired baby may well be disturbed when you move the pillow, in which case you will have to spend an hour or more sitting with him asleep on your lap. Although this is very restricting for you, it is a great deal more relaxing than the alternative of pacing around with your baby over your shoulder. You may also find that you only need to do this after one or two feeds to break the cycle of 'over-tiredness' and from then on your baby will be able to settle himself.

The 'lap' method works extremely well with babies up to the age of about three months. Babies older than this will usually settle best when taken for a long walk in a pram.

Note: It is safe to leave your baby to sleep on his tummy during the day, provided you are around to keep an eye on him. You should *never* leave him lying unattended if you have put him to sleep on his tummy.

Poor weight gain

Most babies have an inbuilt sense of survival and will take as much milk as their body needs. However, some babies are not great eaters and, if left entirely to their own devices, may well take less milk than they need and as a result will not gain the right amount of weight. Sometimes these babies will appear contented and sleep for long periods without showing any signs of needing to feed, making it all too easy to assume that they must be getting enough milk. If your baby's weight gain is fine he clearly is getting enough milk (even if he is taking less milk than other babies of a similar age and weight), but if his weight gain is not good you will need to encourage him to eat more.

If your baby is contented and sleepy (but is not gaining weight) you should:

● Wake him at least every four hours during the day to offer him feeds.
● Make sure that he latches on correctly, so that he can get the milk quickly and easily.
● Keep him awake during feeds by feeding him in a cool room – if necessary, you should also take off some of his clothes so that he is not too warm and cosy.
● Change his nappy when he falls sound asleep, rather than changing it at the start of the feed.

If he is unsettled and fractious (and is not gaining weight), the main reasons for this are likely to be:

● You don't have enough breast milk for him (see Not enough breast milk, page 125).
● You do have enough milk, but you are not feeding him for long enough or frequently enough.
● He is suffering from something simple that is making him too uncomfortable to feed, e.g. wind (see page 35).
● He is allergic/sensitive to something that you are eating (see Milk allergy, page 144).
● He has a medical problem that is making feeding uncomfortable, e.g. thrush (page 153), reflux (page 148) or milk intolerance (page 144).

You will need to go through each point on the checklist above, making the necessary changes to your feeding techniques and your diet, and you should also consult a doctor if you think your baby may have a medical problem. If he is given a clean bill of health and changing the way you feed and wind him makes no difference at all, try offering him extra milk at the end of each feed. This is the quickest and easiest way to discover whether your milk supply is low and whether he needs more milk than your breasts are providing. To establish whether he needs more milk, try offering a top-up bottle at the end of each feed as described below, even if he does not seem to be hungry.

Top-up bottle method

Give your baby a normal-length breast-feed (i.e. feed until you would normally stop) and then straight away offer him extra milk from a bottle, without making any attempt to settle him first. Ideally, you should be offering him breast milk that you have expressed earlier on that day (or got out of the freezer) but if you have no breast milk available you will have to give him formula milk.

- If your baby *always* refuses to take any more milk, this means that you almost certainly do have enough breast milk for him.
- If he *sometimes* takes extra milk, this would indicate that at certain times of the day your breasts may not be making enough milk for him.
- If he always takes extra milk and his weight gain quickly improves, this shows that he was not getting enough milk.

If you discover that the cause of his poor weight gain *is* due to a lack of milk, you will need to see if you can improve your milk supply (see page 126). In the meantime, you should carry on giving your baby the extra milk he needs from a bottle.

If the top-up bottles make no difference to your baby's weight gain, consult your GP or a paediatrician to discuss whether anything needs to be done. Your doctor may feel that your baby is perfectly healthy (see Weight gain, page 75) or he may decide that it is worth carrying out a few tests to see whether there is a medical reason for his not putting on enough weight.

Note: If your baby's stools change from a mustard yellow colour to a dark greenish colour and he is doing less than six wet nappies a day, he is almost certainly getting too little milk and is probably becoming a bit dehydrated. If this happens you must give him more milk.

Milk allergy/food intolerance

When breast-feeding, a mother should be able to eat pretty much whatever she wants as very few foods will affect her baby via the breast milk. However, if you think that your baby *is* being affected by something that you are eating, you may well be right. If he regularly becomes unsettled after you have eaten a certain food, try avoiding that food for a day or two to see whether it makes any difference to his behaviour. If it makes a big difference, you can probably assume that he cannot tolerate you eating that food and you should cut it out of your diet for as long as you are breast-feeding. If your baby is only being affected by one or two foods which commonly affect babies (e.g. citrus fruits, curry or garlic), there is no need to consult a doctor. If, however, your baby is showing signs of lactose intolerance or milk allergy you should see your GP to have a proper diagnosis made.

Lactose intolerance

Lactose is a sugar present in both breast and formula milk, and this is normally broken down by an enzyme in the bowel called lactase, which allows it to be absorbed easily. But if a baby has little or no lactase (this can often result from a bout of gastro-enteritis) he may suffer from excessive wind, abdominal distension and pain, diarrhoea, frothy stools and vomiting. A diagnosis can often be made by a stool test, which will show the stools to be acidic and contain glucose.

Milk allergy

Some babies are allergic to the protein found in milk – this most commonly occurs when a baby is fed formula milk, but some babies are so sensitive that they will also react to breast milk. The symptoms of milk allergy are numerous and can include any of the following – vomiting, colic, rashes and/or swelling around the lips, and eczema. Your baby is also likely to be very hard to feed and settle.

Although it's upsetting if your baby is diagnosed with a milk allergy, you can be comforted by the fact that his symptoms will usually subside quickly once he gets the correct treatment. If you are breast-feeding, your doctor may recommend that you exclude all dairy products from your diet and if you are bottle-feeding, he may prescribe a formula milk that does not contain cow's milk protein.

And the good news is that, given time, nearly all babies will grow out of a milk allergy.

Colic

A baby suffering from colic is not the same as a baby suffering from wind. A 'windy' baby may be very slow to wind but will stop suffering from wind pains as soon as the wind is brought up. A baby suffering from colic, on the other hand, will continue to suffer, regardless of how long you spend winding him. The reason I say this is that, before attempting to treat colic, it is important to establish whether your baby actually has colic or whether he has something else that is making him uncomfortable, e.g. wind, reflux or milk allergy.

Many mothers blame colic whenever their baby is unsettled and sometimes they are right to do so, but frequently they are wrong. Although colic does affect a lot of babies, it is often misdiagnosed (usually by family or friends), so if in doubt consult a doctor.

Colic is a physical discomfort caused by severe spasmodic pain in the abdomen and appears to be just as common in breast-fed babies as in bottle-fed babies. There is a great deal of debate amongst the medical profession as to exactly what causes a baby to suffer from colic, but most doctors would agree with the following:

- Colic could be caused by milk intolerance – breast-feeding mothers who avoid all milk and dairy products will often (but by no means always) find that their baby's colic disappears.
- The pain of colic is caused by a combination of wind and bowel spasms.
- Although the discomfort is associated with wind, wind is not the sole cause of colic (i.e. however thoroughly you wind your baby, the colic will not necessarily go away).
- A colicky baby can be extremely hard to wind.
- For some reason, colic does not necessarily affect a baby after every single feed, so it is possible to have some feeds that end up with the baby falling peacefully asleep without suffering any apparent discomfort.
- Some mothers are (relatively!) lucky and find that their baby only suffers from colic during the day but not at night; some find the reverse, and others are extremely unlucky and find that their baby suffers from colic 24 hours a day.

If your baby appears to be suffering from colic for a large part of the day, it's definitely worth taking him to the doctor to get a proper diagnosis, because you may find that he is suffering from reflux rather than colic. The signs and symptoms of these two conditions are so similar that it will be almost impossible for you to be sure which is causing the problem, whereas your GP can do tests (if necessary) to help him to make a diagnosis.

Signs and symptoms of colic
● The baby does not settle after feeds.
● He cries, draws his legs up to his stomach and appears to be in some pain.
● Winding does not seem to help.
● Putting him back to the breast may stop him crying for a bit (he is comforted by the sucking) but it does not send him to sleep.
● Offering top-up bottles (to make sure he is not hungry) makes no difference to how well he settles after a feed – it may even make the situation worse.
● Nothing stops him crying, other than holding him, rocking him or walking him in a pram.
● The baby starts crying again almost as soon as you stop walking him in the pram.

When a baby shows some, or all, of the above symptoms, it is very easy (and common) for a mother to make the mistake of thinking that he will become easier to manage if she changes from breast-feeding to bottle-feeding. She will often do this because she is worried that her baby is crying because she doesn't have enough milk for him, and thinks that, by giving a bottle, she can be sure that hunger is not the cause of his crying.

The sad fact is that many mothers who do give up breast-feeding find that their baby is equally unsettled on formula milk, and then, to make matters worse, are told by well-meaning friends that their baby would be more settled on breast milk.

It's worth telling these friends (and reminding yourself) that the only reason you gave up breast-feeding was because your baby was *not* settled on breast milk.

Colic usually starts round about the third week and lasts for three to four months before clearing up of its own accord. Although you cannot cure it, there are ways of making it more bearable for both you and your baby.

● Omit any foods from your diet that may be upsetting him.
● Try using the various over-the-counter remedies that are available from the chemist, e.g. gripe water, Infacol or Colief. Some of these can work quite well, so it's worth trying them, but you will often find that what seems to work at some feeds won't work at others.

- Your doctor may prescribe an anti-spasmodic medicine.
- Try using different bottles and teats to see whether this helps – if it does, it is almost certain that your baby has a problem other than colic, e.g. wind.
- Give your baby a dummy to suck on in between feeds.
- Try not to feed him within three hours of the start of the previous feed. If you feed more frequently than this, his colic is likely to become worse – if his tummy is permanently being filled with the cause of his colic (milk) he won't have time to digest one meal before the next is being offered.
- You will usually be able to stop your baby crying by lying him on his tummy on a pillow on your lap, and patting him really firmly on his back for as long as it takes to get him to sleep (see page 139). A baby will find this very soothing and comforting and will usually settle better like this than if you pace around the room with him on your shoulder. It is also more relaxing for you!
- As a last resort, you can nearly always settle a colicky baby by driving him around in your car or by spending long periods wheeling him in a pram. The downside of this is that, not only is it very disruptive to your life, but you may also find that he starts crying again as soon as you stop driving the car or pushing the pram.

If none of the above helps much, it may well be worth looking at alternative medicine. Over the years, I have referred a number of mothers and babies to both homeopaths and cranial osteopaths with fairly impressive results – this may not be the miracle answer to colic, but I do feel it is worth considering when all else fails.

However, it is important to get a proper diagnosis from your GP or a paediatrician before seeking alternative remedies so that you are sure that you (and your therapist) know what you are dealing with.

Coping with a colicky baby is extremely stressful, and knowing that it will only last three or four months seems little comfort. I know this only too well, because my son Richard (my second baby) was a complete nightmare for at least four months and I blame him for me going grey prematurely! During that awful time I have to say that I found it very hard to bond with him and I worried whether I would ever grow to love him as much as his better-behaved sister. However, the good news is that once Richard had recovered from his colic, he became the most lovely, placid baby, and even turned into a delightful teenager! I use this little anecdote to demonstrate that it is not essential to bond with your baby in the first few weeks as you can (and will!) grow to love even the most difficult baby once his endless crying stops.

Note: I have lost count of the number of parents who have consulted me, claiming their baby has terrible colic when this has proved not to be so – in almost every case the problem has been either hunger or reflux. Please do at least rule out these two things before resigning yourself (and your baby) to several months of misery.

Evening colic/evening fretting

It is very common for babies to be unsettled in the evening, usually from about 6pm to 11pm or midnight, and this is often caused by colic which, for some reason, only occurs during this part of the day. Although it is extremely grim to have a baby that needs attention all evening, every evening, you should try to think positively and consider yourself lucky if this is the only time of day that he suffers from colic. Remember, he will normally grow out of it by the time he is about three or four months old.

There's not much you can do to cure a baby who is suffering from evening colic, other than to try the methods described above. However, a mother will often assume that her unsettled baby is suffering from colic when in fact he is either hungry or overtired. It is fairly common for a mother's milk supply to diminish towards the end of the day, with the result that her baby can't always get as much milk in the evening as he does the rest of the day. If you think that you might fall into this category, you should try to improve your milk supply. If you find that you can't and your baby is clearly hungry, your only option is to give him extra milk from a bottle at one of the evening feeds. Many mothers find that giving a bottle at this time of the day does not interfere with milk production during the rest of the 24 hours, but does give the baby the extra milk he needs.

Gastro-oesophageal reflux

This is a condition that affects many babies but frequently goes undiagnosed. Reflux happens when a baby has a weak sphincter muscle at the top of his stomach, allowing the contents of his stomach to go back up into his oesophagus – which gives him the equivalent of acid heartburn. As a result, every time you feed your baby he will suffer pain, and the bigger the feed, the more pain he will suffer. Many people (including doctors) will only consider reflux as a possibility if the baby is bringing up some or most of his feeds, but the fact is that many babies can have severe reflux without ever being seen to vomit up milk. Instead, the milk just goes up and down in the oesophagus, with the stomach acid 'burning' and damaging the delicate tissue which lines the oesophagus.

You should consider reflux if your baby is showing any of the following signs:

- He starts each feed sucking eagerly and well, but then becomes distressed as the feed progresses.
- Typically he will start crying, throwing his head back and arching his back. His whole body may become rigid and it will take several minutes to calm him down.
- He may then refuse to continue feeding, even though he has only taken a small amount of milk.
- He cries after every feed (and usually throughout the feed).
- He will become very distressed if you lie him flat on his back, and he will only stop crying when you hold him upright.
- He brings up more milk after each feed than you would expect with a normal posset.
- He consistently takes small feeds, which last him less than three hours.
- His weight gain is poor but he won't drink more milk.

When a baby is being breast-fed, it can be quite hard to diagnose reflux as many of the above signs and symptoms will occur as a result of breast-feeding problems, rather than the effects of reflux. So, in order to help you make a diagnosis, I suggest that you express your milk and give a few feeds by bottle rather than breast – this way you can see exactly what is happening. The most obvious effect of reflux is that a baby will usually take significantly less milk than he should be taking for his age and size, and this will become very apparent when you can see exactly how much he drinks at each feed. If, for example, your baby needs approximately 180 ml (6 oz) of milk but he will only take 60–90 ml (2–3 oz) before crying, arching his back and refusing to finish the bottle, it will be pretty obvious that he is in pain. As a baby gets older and needs larger amounts of milk, the discrepancy between what your baby *will* take and what he *should* be taking becomes much more obvious.

If you think your baby has reflux, you will need to consult your GP to have the diagnosis confirmed. In obvious cases of reflux, your GP will usually prescribe Infant Gaviscon and, if you are bottle-feeding, he may also recommend you change to a special anti-reflux formula milk. If your baby improves dramatically on Gaviscon, no further treatment or tests should be necessary and he can remain on it until such time as your GP considers that it is no longer needed.

If, however, your baby does not respond to Gaviscon or there is doubt about the diagnosis, your GP may arrange for him to go into hospital for tests. Here, your baby will either be given a barium meal (a special liquid which shows up on x-rays) or he will have a four-hour endoscopy, which measures the acidity at the bottom of the oesophagus. Depending on the results, your baby may then be prescribed an antacid such as Ranitidine or an inhibitor such as Losec, which can stop acid production altogether. Unfortunately, reflux is not always cured overnight and I'm afraid that it occasionally involves many weeks of misery (for both of you) before the right mix of drugs is found and the symptoms of reflux abate. If this does happen, try to comfort yourself with the knowledge that every baby will eventually grow out of reflux, with or without treatment.

Babies with reflux need to be kept upright as much as possible, in order to help keep the milk down in the stomach, so it will help a bit if you:

● Feed your baby in an upright position.
● Keep him sitting upright for at least half an hour after feeds.
● Tilt his cot by propping it up at the head end.

Note: If your baby does not respond well to treatment for reflux and continues to be unable to take in enough milk for his needs, it might be a good idea to start him on solids rather earlier than usual (i.e. well before six months). You could discuss this with your GP or paediatrician.

Within days of my writing this section on reflux, my colleague, Christine Hill, was sent the following letter containing such an accurate description of the agonies suffered by both mother and baby when reflux goes undiagnosed that (with the mother's permission) I felt it worth reproducing for this book. So here it is:

Dear Christine,

This is just a brief note to thank you and your team once again for your help. Although it's been three years since I attended your antenatal classes, I have continued to receive immeasurable assistance from all of you during and after my second pregnancy.

Since his birth, Jonah has been a 'difficult' baby. He often thrashed about and screamed during breast-feeding, never fell asleep on his own (not even at the breast) and had to be carried upright for literally hours each day to stop him from crying. At six weeks, I began to wean him on to bottles, thinking my life would get easier. As I increased the number of bottle-feedings, however, his distress seemed to grow. I thought it was a case of bottle rejection and so stopped breast-feeding entirely.

The feeding problems continued and when he was 10 weeks old I rang Clare to describe the situation to her and she came to my house that same afternoon. After trying to feed Jonah herself for an hour using different teats, etc., she told me that she felt Jonah definitely had a biological problem – reflux or milk allergy or both – and that I needed to see a paediatrician immediately. She explained to me that not all reflux babies vomit.

I did see a paediatrician the next day and Jonah was switched to a non-dairy, non-soy formula and put on Zantac. When he showed no improvement after a week, he was admitted to hospital for pH testing and a barium feed, which showed severe gastro-oesophageal reflux. We are now juggling Cisapride and Losec dosages to try and come up with a combination that will reduce his (and our!) distress.

Words cannot express how grateful I am to Clare. I had felt like the worst mother in the world – not able to feed my son with breast or bottle without ending up in tears. I had described Jonah's behaviour to my GP and two paediatricians, neither of whom picked up on the fact that he had reflux. One paediatrician had said 'maybe it's reflux' but when I responded that Jonah didn't vomit at all, he didn't pursue the point further and explain to me that some babies don't vomit but may still be suffering terribly. Although Jonah's problem is not 'fixed', he has improved on medication and I am in better mental health knowing I am doing all I can for my child.

None of the numerous childcare books I have contain any

information at all about reflux. Many of them do describe 'difficult' babies and urge patience without listing specific symptoms that might in fact indicate a medical problem. I cannot understand how such a relatively common problem goes undiscussed!

In any event, many thanks again to you and Clare for all of the kindness and good sense advice I have received.

Regards,
Ellen

Case History 10
Patti Taylor and Rory and Freya (aged 4 months)

After three months of happy and successful feeding, Patti began weaning her twins on to bottle-feeding in preparation for her return to work. Rory fed well from the outset but Freya would only take small feeds and her weight gain was poor. Patti's GP and several health visitors all assured her that there was no cause for concern and insisted that Rory fed better than his sister simply because 'all babies are different'. They did however suggest trying other bottles and teats to see whether this might help.

At four months, no solution had been found and Patti rang me for an appointment, hoping that I could help get Freya to feed better. Over the phone, Patti described how Freya would take two or three ounces of milk and then suddenly start arching her back, wave her head from side to side and refuse point blank to take any more milk. Although Freya was reasonably settled in between feeds and showing no other symptoms of any significance, I was pretty sure she had reflux and suggested that rather than seeing me, Patti would do better to consult a paediatrician. Patti took some persuasion as she thought this was rather unlikely that I could diagnose reflux over the phone when neither her GP nor any of the health visitors had even mentioned it as a possibility. Nonetheless, she did agree to see a paediatrician, who confirmed the diagnosis and wrote to me saying that Freya did indeed have 'significant symptoms of gastro-oesophageal reflux'. With the correct treatment, Freya gradually started to take more milk at each feed and her weight gain also inproved. Problem solved!

Conclusion: In this case, it was not exactly rocket science to diagnose reflux over the telephone. When a baby should be having about 8 ounces of milk at each feed but will only take two or three, it is much more likely that there is something wrong with the baby than it is for there to be something wrong about the way she is being fed.

Constipation

A breast-fed baby tends to do fewer dirty nappies than a bottle-fed baby because breast milk is so well digested that there is often not much end product. It's perfectly normal for a baby to go three or four days without doing a dirty nappy and, as long as he appears comfortable and his stools are soft, he will not be constipated and will need no treatment. A baby is normally only considered to be constipated if he goes for several days without passing a motion and then produces stools that are hard and pellet-shaped.

If your baby does become constipated, you could try offering him cool, boiled water from a bottle in between feeds. If this doesn't help, adding a teaspoon of brown sugar to the water will often do the trick. Another (and somewhat more effective) remedy for constipation is to give him an ounce or two of diluted prune juice or freshly squeezed orange juice. If his constipation is only temporary and is easily resolved with these home remedies, there is nothing further that needs to be done, but if it persists you should consult a doctor.

Note: Occasionally a baby who appears uncomfortable and colicky and keeps visibly straining to do a dirty nappy, but then produces soft stools, may be suffering from a tight anal sphincter muscle (anal stenosis). Not all GPs are familiar with this condition so he may need to refer you to a paediatrician who will know what to do. Treatment is very simple (it involves gently dilating the sphincter muscle) but it is not something that you should attempt to do yourself.

Thrush

Thrush is a fungal infection caused by the yeast organism *Candida albicans*, which normally lives harmlessly on the skin or in various parts of the body such as the vagina, mouth or bowel. This yeast is usually kept at bay by 'harmless' bacteria and a healthy immune system, but if a mother's immune system is weakened or she is prescribed a course of antibiotics (which will destroy these bacteria) the fungus will flourish and give rise to thrush.

It is fairly common for a mother and/or her baby to get thrush (especially after taking antibiotics) and thrush is easily transmitted between mother and baby and everyone else in the household. So, if either you or your baby gets thrush, you will both need to be treated – you will also need to be meticulous with hygiene and to pay particular attention to sterilising dummies and teats, etc.

Signs of thrush in the mother:

● Cracked and/or sore nipples that don't heal.
● Intense pain in the nipple or the breast (which is not improved by better attachment of the baby to the breast).
● Nipple and/or breast pain that increases during the course of a feed and may continue between feeds.
● The nipple and areola are shiny and pink and may also be itchy.
● Sore nipples that suddenly develop after a period of pain-free breast-feeding.
● Shooting pains in the breast, either during or after feeding – the pain can last up to an hour after feeding.

Signs of thrush in the baby:

● White spots in his mouth.
● A creamy white coating on his tongue, which does not rub off (milk will rub off).
● He keeps pulling off the breast or bottle (because his mouth is sore).
● He may be fretful and difficult to settle.
● He has nappy rash, which is not healing.

If you think you have thrush you should see your GP, who will be able to make a diagnosis and prescribe a suitable treatment. For surface thrush he would normally prescribe Daktarin cream, which you would rub into your nipple after every feed and your baby should be treated with Daktarin oral gel or Nystatin drops, which you apply to his mouth after feeds.

Shooting pains in your breast would indicate that the thrush has entered the milk ducts, in which case you will need oral treatment – a 10-day course of Fluconazole tablets is usually the most effective treatment. Alternatively your GP may prescribe a 14-day course of Nystatin tablets.

You can carry on breast-feeding during treatment and the thrush will usually clear up within a few days – but do be sure to complete the treatment as prescribed by your doctor. Any milk that you have expressed (and possibly frozen) during an episode of thrush should be thrown away, as this may re-infect you and/or your baby.

Note: Acidophilus capsules (available from health food shops or chemists) can help restore healthy bacteria which can keep thrush under control. Eating a small pot of live yoghurt each day will also help reduce your susceptibility to thrush.

Dehydration

Within the first week or so of birth, a baby can become dehydrated very quickly if he is not getting enough milk on a regular basis. This rarely happens when a baby is being bottle-fed as it is pretty obvious if he is not feeding well, but it is far less easy to spot when a baby is breast-feeding. This is because many mothers assume that a baby who is sucking on the breast will always be getting plenty of milk, and they can also be misled into thinking that a baby won't stay asleep if he is hungry and needs feeding. In fact, although most babies *will* cry if they are hungry and won't settle back to sleep until they have had enough milk, others will become drowsy and apathetic and stop waking for feeds. It is therefore important to recognise the signs of dehydration so you can take prompt action.

Your baby may be becoming dehydrated if:

- He keeps crying for a feed but then falls asleep after only a few sucks at the breast.
- He becomes sleepy and listless and stops waking for feeds.
- He goes for more than six hours without doing a wet nappy.
- His urine smells strong.
- He has a sunken fontanelle (the soft bit on the top of his skull where the bones have not yet fused).

If you think your baby is becoming dehydrated, you should try to get more milk into him as soon as possible. If you can't get him to feed more at the breast, you should express your milk (or open a carton of formula if you can't express any milk) and offer it to him in a bottle. As a rule of thumb, I have found that a baby who is able to drink at least 30 ml (1 oz) of milk is usually fine but if he takes less than this he is probably sufficiently dehydrated to require hospital treatment.

If, however, you were using an Avent teat, it is worth first trying to feed him again using a different teat (e.g. Nuk) as I often find that a baby will feed better from a softer teat. If this doesn't do the trick you should ring your local hospital or GP to discuss the situation.

If your baby is admitted to hospital, you can expect him to stay in for one or two days, during which time he may need to be fed by tube or intravenous infusion. The hospital staff should also make sure that breast-feeding is fully and properly established before discharging you both home.

Having a baby admitted to hospital suffering from dehydration is not only extremely distressing but can also knock a mother's confidence in breast-feeding – it is therefore very important to get all the support and reassurance that you need to encourage you to continue. I also think it is worth offering top-up bottles for the first few feeds after you get home so that you can see whether your baby is getting all the milk he needs.

Refusing bottles

Most baby books gloss over the issue of bottle rejection, suggesting that it is a problem that can be solved simply by offering the baby a bottle on a regular basis and waiting for him to take to it in his own time. If only it were this simple! Unfortunately, the reality is that a large number of babies will become more (rather than less) resistant to the bottle as the weeks go and using this 'softly, softly' approach rarely works.

I am regularly consulted by mothers whose baby won't take a bottle and most of them have very legitimate reasons (see Introducing a bottle, page 94) for needing to introduce bottle feeds. Because I see at first hand the trauma and distress that is created when a baby rejects the bottle, I regard this as a very important issue that needs addressing – I do *not* think it is cruel to teach a baby to feed from a bottle. Nor do I see any evidence that a baby suffers any lasting trauma when he is persuaded (against his will) to take a bottle, and the letters and phone calls I receive from the mothers would confirm this.

I don't know why some babies are so reluctant to feed from a bottle, but I can only assume that it's because they are used to a nice soft, warm breast and find that a rubbery teat does not compare favourably. I also get the impression that some babies are frightened of the bottle, either because the milk flows so differently and/or because they have choked on one when it was first given and immediately developed an aversion to this method of feeding.

Regardless of the reason why your baby is rejecting the bottle, it's always very difficult to deal with and the older the baby becomes, the harder it is to resolve. It is much easier to persuade a baby under the age of three months to take a bottle than it is to persuade an older baby, and for this reason I do recommend that you tackle the problem head on as soon as it arises. In other words, if your baby first rejects the bottle when he is quite young, it is not a good idea to bury your head in the sand and hope the problem will go away. It won't! Instead, you should make a concerted effort there and then to get him to take a bottle and if necessary set aside a 24-hour period to do it in.

There are no easy answers to this problem and what works with one baby will not necessarily work with another. However, the general principle involved is to get the baby to realise that there is something nice in the bottle! Hopefully you can achieve this by reading on.

There are two main types of bottle-rejecting babies:

● The ones who will happily sit for a good 10 minutes or so rolling the teat around under their tongue and from side to side in their mouth before deciding playtime is over and they want to be fed – at which point they start screaming.
● Those who go ballistic as soon as they see the bottle or as soon as the teat touches their lips. With these babies you will feel you have lost the battle before you even get past square one.

With both types of babies, the key to success is to try and get the baby to suck on the bottle by instinct (rather than desire) and then to make sure that he gets the milk quickly and easily and that he doesn't choke on it. To achieve this, you need to distract him so he doesn't notice you putting the bottle in his mouth, and then you hope that his automatic response is to start sucking. When this works, the mother is so amazed, that she doesn't know whether to shed tears of joy or tears of frustration that the problem has been solved so easily! However, many babies are not this easily duped and for these a much more robust approach is required! You may need to spend at least an hour trying to get him to feed, he may cry a lot and you should also be prepared for it to take a full 24 hours before he accepts the bottle. I usually find I can get a baby to accept the bottle without too many tears, but even the ones who do cry are usually happily smiling at the end of the session – even if they are still refusing to feed and are still hungry.

So, please don't worry if your baby resists and cries a lot, and be assured that he will come to no harm and will certainly harbour no grudge against you.

As some babies will hold out for the full 24 hours, you should only embark on this robust approach if you are determined to see it through – if you give in within this time all your efforts will have been wasted and your baby will be even harder to convert to the bottle next time you try.

These are my tips:

- Set aside a 24-hour period during which time you will only offer your baby the bottle, i.e. no breast and no solid food.
- Try to choose a day when someone is around to help and support you, but you should be the one to feed your baby. Babies don't seem to react to the breast being so near (and yet so far!) and will usually feel more secure when handled by you.
- Don't give your baby anything at all to eat or drink for at least four hours before attempting to offer him a bottle. He must be hungry and want to feed.
- Have a variety of teats and bottles to hand and experiment to see whether he appears to prefer one more than another. Most babies prefer a very soft teat – I have most success using Playtex or Nuk.
- Start off using a teat with a *very* fast flow so that milk pours into your baby's mouth without him needing to suck. I usually create my own fast-flow teat by using a hot needle to make the existing hole bigger- for this you need to use a latex teat. A fast-flow teat tends to work well with babies who scream as soon as the teat goes in their mouth, before they have even had a chance to realise that they are being given milk.
- It doesn't seem to matter what you put in the bottle (it's the bottle your baby is objecting to rather than its contents), but if you can use expressed breast milk at least you will know that your baby likes what you are offering him. If you can't manage to express enough milk (and/or get discouraged by the wastage if your baby won't drink it), formula milk is the next best thing to use. Babies tend to prefer formula milk to plain water, especially when they are hungry.

- Heat the milk so that it is as warm as possible, but not so warm that you risk burning your baby's mouth – breast-fed babies seem to like the milk to be very warm.
- Sit your baby bolt upright on your lap when you feed so that he won't choke and panic if the milk flow is too fast for him – you should *not* have him lying in your arms in the position you would adopt if you were breast-feeding him.
- Before putting the teat in your baby's mouth, try to attract his attention by waving rattles, etc., and then quickly put the teat in his mouth before he realises what you're doing. The theory behind this is that a baby will automatically suck on anything that goes in his mouth, provided he has not decided in advance that he doesn't want to. You may need to get someone else to wave the rattles, but if no one else is around you could try sitting with him in front of the television or anything else that will distract him.
- If your baby starts crying while you are trying to feed him, don't be put off – keep the teat in his mouth as this is the only way you will ever get him to suck on it. If you keep taking the teat out of his mouth, you will only upset him further and he will never learn that there is nice milk in the bottle.
- If he continues to cry, stand up and walk around with him while still keeping the teat in his mouth – many babies stop crying when you do this.
- If/when he starts sucking really strongly, you will probably need to change him on to a slightly slower teat to prevent him being overwhelmed by the milk flow.
- You may need to spend a minimum of one hour battling with your baby, but don't let his tears put you off. It is not cruel to do this to him and, if you have a deadline (i.e. you have to go back to work) he *must* learn to take his feeds from a bottle, however traumatic it seems at the time.
- If your baby falls into an exhausted sleep without having taken any milk, let him sleep and then start the whole process again when he wakes up. Keep on doing this until he realises that it is the bottle or nothing and decides he needs milk more than he needs your breast!

You can use the same bottle of milk for up to one-and-a-half hours, reheating it as often as is necessary to keep it at an attractive temperature for him. Any milk that is left in the bottle after this time should be thrown away and a fresh bottle should be used for the next feeding attempt.

Most of the babies I deal with need only one session to get them happily on to the bottle and the majority of these continue to feed well from then on – it is quite unusual for a mother to find that her baby refuses the next feed after a successful feed with me. If, however, the baby does not accept the bottle at that first session, he will almost certainly take to the bottle at one of the subsequent feeds within the next 24 hours – so don't give up too soon.

For peace of mind, you might prefer to check with your GP before embarking on what could be a 24-hour marathon, but a normal healthy baby should come to no harm going without food for this long. After all, if you went under a bus tomorrow, your baby would not starve to death – he *would* take a bottle if that were his only option! I am aware that this sounds very harsh, but almost every week I see mothers for whom bottle rejection has become a real issue. Many of their babies are refusing to feed from a bottle even though they are clearly hungry and underweight, and in other cases the mother is becoming desperate because she is due to start back at work and feels she can't leave a baby who won't feed without her. I always feel that the sooner this issue is resolved the better and I also see how life is transformed for the whole family once the baby accepts the bottle. Everyone is happier.

Once your baby is happily taking a bottle, it is up to you to decide whether you can risk combining bottle-feeding and breast-feeding, or whether you feel that it's better to give up breast-feeding completely at this point. Most babies are perfectly happy to do a combination of the two, but I do occasionally come across some who revert to refusing a bottle as soon as they rediscover the breast. The choice (and risk) is yours!

This is a sample of just some of the letters that I have received, showing that most babies are happy taking a mixture of breast and bottle:

Dear Clare,
Thank you so much for your invaluable help in a moment of crisis! Molly now doesn't care where her food comes from as long as she gets it, and doesn't look as if she ever missed a meal!

Many thanks,
Sarah

. . . .

Dear Clare,

Thank you so much for your much-needed assistance. Alice has never looked back. She is happily taking both my milk and the formula from the bottle. It will make my life much easier.

Yours,
Georgina

. . . .

Dear Clare,

Thank you for enabling me to resume a slightly more normal existence by converting my totally breast-fed Tilly on to a bottle. She appears to be more contented and certainly is now gaining more weight. I can also add, she even becomes excited once the bottle is in view!

Kindest regards,
Rebecca

Baby in special care baby unit

If your baby is admitted to the special care baby unit you can, and should, still be able to breast-feed him, even if he is not initially able to feed directly from your breast. A baby needing special care will benefit greatly by being fed breast milk (rather than formula) and it will also help you to feel involved with your baby's care and well-being.

The midwives looking after your baby will discuss feeding with you and will let you know whether he is able to breast-feed, or whether he temporarily needs to be fed by other means, e.g. by intravenous infusion or with a naso-gastric tube.

If he *is* unable to breast-feed, you will need to express your milk regularly using a breast pump – to maintain your milk supply and provide milk for your baby. All special care baby units have the full equipment necessary for expressing and you will be shown how to use it. You will also be advised on how often you need to express – this should be at least every four hours day and night in order to keep your milk supply going. Any milk you express can be given to your baby at subsequent feeds or can be frozen and kept for him to have at a later date.

Don't worry if your baby can't breast-feed initially, as this should not prevent him sucking on the breast at a later date. Virtually all babies will happily revert to the breast (even if they've been bottle-fed for several weeks) once they are well enough to do so. My own son was born a month early and spent the first 10 days of his life on a ventilator (his lungs were not fully developed), but he had no problems at all in rushing to the breast as soon as it was offered to him! I also know of many other babies who have equally happily gone on to the breast even after many weeks of being tube-fed or bottle-fed.

If you decide that you don't want to breast-feed at all, you will need to discuss with the medical staff what, if anything, should be done to stop your milk coming in. Some doctors are happy to prescribe tablets to dry up the milk supply, while others prefer to let nature take its course and leave it to stop of its own accord.

If the latter is the case, your milk will come in around Day 3 or 4, your breasts will rapidly become engorged and painful, and you may develop mastitis (see page 119). They will remain like this for a minimum of two days before they soften up and stop producing milk. During this time you will need to wear a good supporting bra and you may need to take mild painkillers (e.g. paracetamol) as well.

9 Bottle-feeding

I have devoted an entire chapter to bottle-feeding, mainly because I have been asked so many questions on the subject that I have come to realise that the average mother does not know as much about it as she could, or should, know. I have also found that many shop assistants are not very well-informed when it comes to discussing the merits of the different types of bottles, teats, etc., and may not be able to give you the information you need on subjects such as how to sterilise the equipment. I hope that this chapter will cover pretty much everything you could ever want or need to know about bottle-feeding. Bottle-feeding is not just a question of throwing any formula into any bottle and giving it to your baby at any time of day or night!

Equipment

When it comes to bottle-feeding your baby you will discover that while there is some equipment that is essential (e.g. bottles!) there is also some that you can do without. For example, you don't need to buy a steriliser, as it's perfectly possible to make do with something like an old ice-cream container for sterilising your bottles. The main advantage in buying all the correct kit is that it is designed to make the sterilisation and preparation of bottles as easy as possible. The downside of buying more than you need is that it will clutter up your kitchen and will then need to be stored until the next baby. For this reason, I suggest that you start off by getting in the barest minimum and seeing how you get on (on the basis that you can always buy more things as and when you need them). If you can, it's a good idea to decide which brand of products you like the best and then stick to buying within that particular range, as the products will be designed to interact with each other. For example, the Avent bottles will clip on to the Avent breast pump and will also pack perfectly into the Avent steam steriliser, but the Avent bottle will not, for example, fit on a Medela pump.

You will need:

- six 250 ml (8 oz) bottles
- six teats
- a bottle brush
- a steriliser
- a plastic jug
- a plastic knife or spatula
- sterilising solution or tablets (if you are sterilising using the soaking method).

Note: If you begin bottle-feeding when your baby is having fewer than six feeds a day, you will not need six bottles. You need enough bottles to make up feeds for a 24-hour period, with perhaps one extra bottle as a spare.

Bottles

There are many different types of bottle on the market and they all work! However, each manufacturer will give reasons as to why theirs is the best (e.g. by claiming to reduce the amount of air your baby will take in during feeds), so it can be quite hard to know which one is the best to buy. Despite all the claims, I have not found that any one bottle 'works' substantially better than another but I have noticed that babies that are poor feeders will sometimes feed better if you change to a different type of bottle and teat – if, for example, your baby is feeding badly or 'messily' it is well worth experimenting to see what suits him best. As many of the anti-colic bottles are very fiddly both to assemble and clean, I would only opt for these if you have established that your baby cannot feed well from a more basic bottle.

Teats

Teats come in all shapes and sizes, with variable flow rates (slow, medium and fast), and are made from either silicone or latex. Silicone is more durable but latex has the advantage of you being able to enlarge the size of the hole if your baby needs a faster flow.

As with bottles, I think the type of teat you use makes little difference to how much air your baby takes in during feeds, so it's really down to what suits him best. You will need to discover for yourself whether he likes a slow-, medium- or fast-flow teat but, as a general rule, the medium-flow is a good one to start with. Regardless of his age, it should take your baby approximately 20 minutes to empty the bottle (because a bigger baby feeds more 'strongly' so feeds don't take longer) so if he takes much longer than this you could try using a faster-flow teat. If you are using latex teats you won't need to buy new ones as you can speed up the flow of milk by enlarging the existing hole. All you have to do is heat a pin over a naked flame until it is glowing red hot (use a clothes peg to hold the pin so you don't get burnt!) and then quickly insert the hot pin into the hole. The more you do this, the bigger the hole will become and the faster the milk will flow. Unfortunately, you can't do this with silicone teats. If, on the other hand, your baby is emptying the bottle too quickly, you should change to a slower teat to allow him more time to enjoy his feed.

Sterilisers

The main thing to look out for when choosing a steriliser is that it will hold the bottles you are using, as each steriliser is designed to take a certain shape of bottle. For example, the Avent steriliser is designed to be packed with short wide bottles, rather than with tall narrow ones. You will still be able to sterilise other manufacturers' bottles in an Avent steriliser, but they may not pack in as efficiently.

Sterilising

Most mothers are aware of the importance of sterilising everything, but few fully understand why it needs to be done. I am always being asked questions about this and find that once I explain the reasoning behind it, mothers become much more confident about their own ability to decide what needs sterilising, how often, and when they can stop sterilising altogether.

The main reasons why you need to sterilise are:

- Young babies are very susceptible to germs.
- Milk is a perfect medium in which germs can multiply.
- Sterilising is the best way to ensure that germs are destroyed.

Although health professionals usually recommend that you sterilise all your baby's feeding equipment for a minimum of six months, it is in fact safe to use something that has not been sterilised (e.g. a nipple shield) provided you have washed it properly. This makes obvious sense when you appreciate that not everything that goes into your baby's mouth has to be sterilised (your breast or finger, for example). However, anything that is not being sterilised does have to be washed carefully and as often as is necessary. You would not (I hope!) allow your baby to suck on your finger without first washing your hands but, having washed your hands once, you would not need to wash them again until you did something that might contaminate them, such as a nappy change. You would also know to wash your hands much more thoroughly after, say, handling raw chicken than you would after preparing sandwiches or other such food.

A similar principle is involved when it comes to other things that go in your baby's mouth. For example, a dummy that falls out of your baby's mouth into his cot can be put straight back into his mouth, but a dummy that falls on to a dirty street should not be used again until it has been sterilised (or washed very thoroughly if you don't have a spare one to hand). **Putting the dummy in your own mouth and sucking on it does not make it germ-free and safe to go back in the baby's mouth.** Bottles will need sterilising, however, because milk is a perfect medium in which bacteria can multiply. If a bottle is not completely clean when you fill it with milk, any bacteria it contains will start multiplying at such a rate that by the time you give the feed there may be enough present to give your baby a tummy upset. A minor tummy upset won't do him much harm (although it can be unpleasant), but if there's a particularly nasty bug in the bottle, your baby could contract a severe case of gastro-enteritis and might need to be admitted to hospital. Obviously, it is best to avoid this, which is why it's better to be safe than sorry and to sterilise all your bottles. However, if you do need a bottle in a hurry and don't have time to sterilise it, there is unlikely to be a problem if you wash the bottle thoroughly, fill it with milk and use it immediately. Any bacteria that might be left inside would not have a chance to multiply to a dangerous level in such a short time.

Everything you wash (but are not planning to sterilise) should either be dried with a freshly laundered drying-up cloth or paper towel, or left to drip-dry on a clean rack. If you use a grubby drying-up cloth or put the washing to drain on a dirty work surface, you will immediately contaminate the items and, in doing so, make them unsafe to use.

In the USA, many mothers put all their baby-feeding equipment in the dishwasher and do not sterilise any of it. This is less safe to do here, because dishwashers in the UK wash at a lower temperature than they do in the USA.

Washing before sterilising

Sterilising is not a substitute for washing, so everything must be washed thoroughly before you sterilise it. Bottles, teats, etc., should be rinsed out in cold water immediately after use and can then be left to one side until you are ready to wash them.

Fill a sink with hot soapy water and then wash each bottle really thoroughly, using a bottle-brush inside and out, making sure that you brush around the ridges of the bottle and its screw top. Teats can be washed by squirting a bit of neat washing-up liquid into them and then giving them a good squidge around (both inside and out) using your fingers. An alternative to washing-up liquid is salt, but this tends to be a bit more fiddly to use when your hands are wet.

Everything should then be rinsed with clean water and put straight into the steriliser – you do not need to dry them first. The bottle brush does not need to be sterilised, but should be kept in a clean place, e.g. in a jam jar (which you should also wash regularly).

Different ways of sterilising

There are four ways of sterilising: steaming, microwaving, using a sterilising solution (the soaking method) or boiling in water.

Steam sterilisers. This is probably the most popular method of sterilising as it is so quick and easy (it takes approximately 10 minutes) and has the additional benefit of not involving any chemicals. Each steriliser will come with clear instructions for its use.

Note: It may be worth having a small bottle of sterilising fluid to take away with you when you visit friends or family – you will find this is much more practical than carting around all your sterilising equipment.

Microwave sterilisers. These work in the same way as steam sterilisers apart from the fact that you will need a microwave oven to operate it. It's worth bearing this in mind when buying one, because if you plan to go and stay with family or friends on a regular basis, your steriliser will be useless if they do not have a microwave oven.

Sterilising solution (the soaking method). This is a good method if you are mainly breast-feeding, and only need to sterilise the occasional bottle, dummy, etc., as it won't be worth cluttering up your kitchen with a big sterilising unit. You can use any non-metallic container (e.g. a plastic jug, ice-cream container or Pyrex bowl), which you fill with ordinary tap water and a measure of sterilising solution. All items to be sterilised must be fully submerged in the sterilising solution (you may need to use a saucer to weigh them down) and then left to soak for a minimum of two hours. Sterilising fluid or tablets can be bought from any chemist and come with full instructions for their use. The main disadvantage of this method is that the solution needs to be changed every 24 hours and the chemicals are fairly tough on your hands, which can become dry and chapped.

The boiling method. Very few mothers use this nowadays although it works perfectly well, especially in an emergency if you have nothing else to hand. All items needing to be sterilised must be immersed in water and boiled for at least 10 minutes – they will then remain sterile for as long as you keep them in the water with the lid of the saucepan on. But if you lift the lid, sneeze into the saucepan, and then put the lid back on, the contents will no longer be sterile!

Different types of formula milk

There are many different brands of formula milk on the market and they all seem to work pretty well! I have not found any one to be better than another, so I tend to suggest that mothers should either choose a formula that is recommended to them by a health care professional, or one that their friends currently think is the best. Most mothers buy tins of powdered milk formula (as this is the most economical option) but ready-made formula can be bought from most chemists and supermarkets in small cartons. These cartons can be stored at room temperature and can then be poured straight into a bottle and fed to the baby without warming it. Any milk left in the carton should then be stored in the fridge in accordance with the instructions on the pack. These cartons are ideal for travelling or for a breast-fed baby who only needs the occasional formula milk top-up feed.

If the formula you choose doesn't appear to agree with your baby (i.e. he sicks quite a lot of it up, he becomes 'mucusy' or he just won't drink much), don't keep changing brands as there might be another cause for his symptoms. Discuss the symptoms with your doctor and take his advice. If there is a strong family history of allergies, it might be wise to consider using a hypo-allergenic formula, but you should also discuss this with your doctor first – it's not a good idea to label your baby as 'allergic' without first getting a proper diagnosis.

These special formulas are usually more expensive than the ordinary ones, but you may well be able to get it on prescription if this is what your doctor recommends. Whichever formula you choose, make sure that you buy one that is suitable for your baby's age. Start with the 'lightest' one and graduate to milk for the 'hungrier baby', if or when your baby appears to need it. Contrary to what some mothers think, milk for the hungrier baby is not more fattening than ordinary milk – it is merely harder to digest and therefore stays longer in the baby's stomach, leaving him feeling contented for longer.

Each tin of formula milk comes with full instructions on how to make up the feeds and will also have a chart with feeding guidelines telling you roughly how much milk your baby will need according to his age and weight. Bear in mind, however, that this is only an approximate guide so, as long as his weight gain is good, it won't matter whether he is drinking more or less than the chart recommends.

Note: If you think your baby has a milk allergy, you should not switch to a goats' milk formula, as almost all babies who are allergic to cows' milk are also allergic to goats' milk. Goats' milk is not easier for a baby to digest and it is also considered to be unsuitable for very young babies because the level of proteins is too concentrated.

Making up the feeds

Ideally, you should get into the habit of making up all the feeds at the same time each day (it is quicker and more efficient to do this) rather than doing each individual bottle as and when you need it.

If you can, try to set aside one part of the work surface in your kitchen exclusively for preparing the bottles and make sure you keep this area scrupulously clean.

When you are ready to make up the feeds you should:

● Rinse out the kettle, fill it with water (taken from the cold water tap) and bring it to the boil.

- Allow the water to cool for about 10 minutes (so that the water is still hot, but not boiling).
- Wash your hands, take the bottles out of the steriliser and stand them on a clean work surface.
- Fill the bottles with the correct amount of water, i.e. 180 ml (6 oz) of water if you want to make up 180 ml (6 oz) of milk.
- Add the milk powder to the water, first checking the tin for instructions as to how much powder to add (it is usually one level scoop of powder per ounce of water).
- Dissolve the powder by putting the tops back on the bottles and giving them a really good shake.
- Sterilise any jugs used for making up the feeds. Make sure you use a sterile plastic fork or knife to stir and dissolve the powder.
- Put bottles straight into the fridge, even though they will be quite hot (the sooner you cool the milk down, the sooner you will stop germs multiplying if you have failed to sterilise the bottles correctly).

Do not:

- Use mineral water as this is designed for adults, not babies (unless the bottle specifically states that it is suitable for babies).
- Use water that has been softened (i.e. if you have a water softener in your house).
- Boil the water more than once as this concentrates the chemicals in the water.
- Use milk that is more than 24 hours old – all old milk must be thrown away.
- Put a half-finished bottle of milk in the fridge to use again later in the day. Bottles should be kept in the fridge (or in a freezer bag if you are travelling) until you are ready to use them.

Note: It is only necessary to use bottled water in countries where the water is not considered to be safe to drink and you should always boil the water, regardless of whether you are using tap or bottled water.

Warming the milk?
It is perfectly all right to feed your baby with cold milk taken straight from the fridge and babies that are used to this from the outset are normally perfectly happy. However, I feel that it is nicer for babies to

be given warm milk (especially during the winter months) and so I suggest that you do warm the milk before offering it to your baby. You can heat the milk either by standing the bottle in a jug of hot water or by using a thermostatically controlled bottle warmer available from most baby shops. Current advice is that a microwave should not be used to heat either breast or formula milk as there is some evidence that this will change the composition of the milk.

All the above methods work perfectly well, but it's essential that you check the temperature of the milk before giving it to your baby. You can test this by shaking a few drops on to the back of your hand – they should feel warm but not hot. A baby's mouth is very sensitive and easily burnt so, if in doubt, it's far better to give the milk slightly too cold than slightly too hot.

If your baby's bedroom is a long way from the kitchen, you can save time at night by taking a vacuum flask of hot water (to heat the bottle) upstairs with you when you go to bed. The milk can also be taken upstairs and kept cool in a freezer bag.

It's well worth varying the temperature of the milk you give your baby, as occasionally babies can become very fussy and start refusing the milk if it is not always at exactly the temperature they are used to.

Giving the feed

Regardless of whether you are breast-feeding or bottle-feeding, it's always worth making sure that you find somewhere comfortable to sit so that you can both relax and enjoy the feed. When bottle-feeding, you need to hold your baby in a slightly more upright position than you would if you were breast-feeding – this ensures that he won't choke on the milk (if it flows too fast) and also helps the wind to come up as he feeds. You should also make sure that you hold the bottle in such a way that the teat is always completely filled with milk so that he does not take in too much air. You may find it more comfortable and less tiring to put a pillow under your arm to help to support your baby while you feed him – even a small baby can place quite a strain on your arm if you have to hold him for a 20-minute (or longer) feed.

Babies normally love their bottle-feed and like to suck fairly slowly and steadily, so that each feed lasts approximately 20 minutes. If the feed is over much more quickly than this, your baby will lose one of the pleasures in life! It is equally important that a feed doesn't take much longer than 20 minutes because, if this happens, a baby can get tired and may then fall asleep before he has drunk all the milk he needs. You may need to experiment a bit to find out which teat and which milk flow works best for him.

Winding your baby

When it comes to winding, all babies are different, with some needing very frequent winding and others only needing winding once or twice during a feed. It is only by trial and error that you will establish what suits your baby and he will come to no harm if you wind him too much or too little (although he might get irritated if you get it too wrong!) A baby will normally let you know when he needs to be winded (by stopping feeding and/or crying), so to begin with you can allow him to carry on sucking for as long as he wants and only wind him when he stops feeding or seems to be uncomfortable. However, if you find your baby brings up a lot of milk when you wind him, try winding him earlier and see whether this suits him better. It doesn't matter if he brings up a lot of milk but if he brings up too much you may then need to replace some of it by feeding him a bit more – this can become rather time-consuming. You need to spend only a minute or two winding your baby during the feed, even if he doesn't bring up any wind in this time. But you should wind him much more thoroughly at the end, because you will find that he is unlikely to settle down to sleep if he is still feeling uncomfortable with wind (see Winding, page 35).

How much milk to offer

It's impossible to be precise about exactly how much milk should be given as all babies' needs differ. However, as a rough guide, most babies under the age of four months will need approximately 150 ml of milk per kg of body weight (or 2½–3 oz per lb) during each 24-hour period. To work out how much your baby will need at each feed, you will need to divide the total amount of milk he needs by the number of feeds he is having.

Metric   *For a 3 kg baby on six feeds a day, you would multiply 3 kg by 150 ml = 450 ml. Divided by six feeds = 75 ml per feed.*

Imperial   *For a 7 lb baby on seven feeds a day, you should multiply 7 lb by 3 oz = 21 oz. Divided by seven feeds = 3 oz per feed. (For ease of maths, I have multiplied by 3 oz, rather than by 2½ oz.)*

This is only a rough guide, so don't worry if your baby takes slightly more or less than this. You should always make up a bit more than you think he needs so that if he is particularly hungry at one feed he can have more, and there should always be a small amount of milk left in the bottle at the end of each feed. That way, you can be fairly sure that he has stopped feeding because he has had enough milk, rather than because there was no more milk available to him. The best way to judge whether your baby is getting the right amount of milk is to weigh him regularly – if he is putting on too much or too little weight you can adjust the amount of milk that you offer him.

Although a bottle-fed baby tends to take pretty much the same amount of milk at each feed, you can still expect your baby's appetite to vary a little from feed to feed, so don't worry if he doesn't always finish the bottle. In fact, you shouldn't try and make him finish it when he has clearly had enough, as this is likely to make him put on more weight than he should.

Of course, if you notice that your baby doesn't last as long in between feeds whenever he has taken significantly less milk than usual, it would be sensible to try to persuade him to take a little bit more milk and see whether this improves things.

If you have a very hungry baby who is not satisfied for long in between feeds, you could try changing him on to a formula milk designed for the hungrier baby and see whether this helps.

Baby bottle tooth decay

Baby bottle tooth decay is a serious condition that can destroy your child's primary teeth when they start coming through at about six months. It occurs when teeth are frequently exposed to liquids containing sugar, such as formula milk, breast milk, cow's milk and fruit juice. When bottle-feeding, the milk pools around your baby's teeth providing food for decay-producing bacteria, which then form acids that damage the tooth enamel. To stop this happening, it is important to start teaching your baby to take some of his feeds from a special cup at about six months and to stop bottle-feeding completely by the age of one year.

Excessive weight gain

A lot of mothers think that it's impossible to overfeed a baby because he will always stop feeding when he's had enough. Unfortunately, this is not true. In fact, it tends to be easier to overfeed a bottle-fed baby than a breast-fed baby, possibly because formula milk is so much more readily available than breast milk. Also, the average mother will often worry if her baby doesn't finish the bottle and may try to persuade him to take more – especially if it's the last feed of the day and she wants a good night's sleep! As breast-feeding mothers can't see how much milk their babies have had, they are less likely to try to persuade him to carry on feeding once he stops. If you regularly give your baby an extra ounce or two more milk than he actually needs, he will almost certainly put on too much weight.

If your baby is overweight:

● See Weight gain, page 75.
● Do not persuade him to finish bottles.
● Try using a slower teat if your baby finishes his bottles too quickly and then cries for more milk.
● Try distracting him, when he's finished the bottle, by walking around with him for a bit – this will allow time for the message to get through from his stomach to his brain to say he's full!
● Try changing him on to a formula milk for the hungrier baby.
● Try mixing his milk with one less scoop of powder (this will still make him feel full, but he will be getting fewer calories). **Never** make the feed more concentrated by adding extra powder.

If your baby continues to pile on the weight despite your efforts to reduce his milk intake, you should probably just relax and accept that you have a very hungry baby who is temporarily going through a growth spurt. You should offer him as much milk as it takes to keep him happy and contented, and you may need to start him on solids before six months. You will probably find that solid food will satisfy him more than milk, while providing fewer calories. Ask your GP's advice on this.

Poor weight gain (when bottle-feeding)

Some babies fail to put on enough weight but are happy and contented, while others fail to put on weight and are clearly both unhappy and hungry. If your baby is happy and contented, his failure to put on weight may be due to his own individual make-up and not anything to worry about. A baby like this will often have a growth spurt and suddenly put on a lot of weight in a short space of time.

But if your baby is not happy and settled and appears to be hungry, you need to discover why this is, and do something about it.

The two main reasons why a baby fails to put on enough weight are:

1. He is not being offered enough milk.
2. He *is* being offered enough milk but he won't drink it.

The first thing to check is whether you are offering your baby enough milk. I know this sounds obvious, but I have seen many a mother who is consistently giving too little milk to her baby and is then absolutely amazed when I point out that her baby is hungry! I find that this most often happens when a baby is born prematurely and the mother is given strict initial guidelines on how much milk her baby should have at each feed, but isn't then told that she should increase the amount as he gets older.

Start by offering your baby extra milk at each feed, but if he doesn't want, or can't manage, larger feeds, try introducing an extra feed during the day to see whether this suits him better. This won't necessarily solve the problem either because you may find that he then takes less milk at the next feed – you will need to experiment to see what happens. If he happily takes more milk and his weight gain improves, you have got the answer to your problem and will need do nothing more.

If you are offering your baby plenty of milk but he won't drink it, he may have a minor medical problem that is making feeding uncomfortable. The most common reason why a baby won't drink enough milk for his needs is physical discomfort caused by conditions such as colic, milk intolerance, reflux or a tight anal sphincter muscle. From a health point of view, none of these conditions is serious and, as most babies will grow out of them in time, it is not essential to do anything.

However, if the condition is severe enough to have a huge impact either on your baby's weight gain or to make life extremely unpleasant for your baby (and you), it is worth investigating to see whether anything can be done. You should take him to your doctor to get him checked over. If he can't find anything wrong, you may just have to battle on and hope that his appetite will pick up. Some babies are not great fans of milk and only really get to grips with eating when you start them on solids.

Note: Some GPs are extremely sympathetic when presented with a crying mother and baby. Others aren't, and don't fully appreciate how desperate a mother can feel if her baby won't feed and is then awake and crying for large parts of the day and night. If your GP falls into the latter category and takes the view that nothing can or needs to be done, it's worth seeking another opinion if you're still worried. Remember, not all GPs have enough experience with babies to diagnose conditions such as reflux or anal stenosis (some haven't even heard of the latter). I know of several mothers who, having been dismissed by their GPs as worrying about nothing, have sought a second opinion – in each case the mother has seen a paediatrician who has diagnosed a problem, treated it successfully and made life infinitely better for both mother and baby.

The most important thing is to see a doctor in whom you have confidence (whether it's your GP or a paediatrician) so that if he tells you not to worry about your baby's poor weight gain, you do stop worrying!

10 Other issues

Tongue-tie

Tongue-tie is a condition (officially known as ankyloglossia) that affects a small number of babies and is often hereditary. There is no means of prevention so it is simply bad luck if your baby is affected by this, but for the majority of babies tongue-tie causes little or no problems and will therefore need no treatment. Tongue-tie occurs when the membrane (the frenulum) that attaches the tongue to the floor of the mouth is too short and tight and extends too far towards the tip of the tongue. This prevents the tongue from moving freely and as a result can sometimes make it difficult, or even impossible, for your baby to breast-feed. If this happens, you should consult a doctor with a view to getting the tongue-tie clipped.

Signs of severe tongue-tie:

- The tip of your baby's tongue does not protrude past the lower gum line.
- Your baby cannot move his tongue from side to side.
- His tongue curls under (rather than upwards) when he cries
- There is a V-shaped notch at the tip of his tongue
- Your baby is finding it hard to latch on and 'milk' your breast efficiently.
- Breast-feeding is painful for you.

Releasing a tongue-tie is normally a quick and painless procedure that can be done without any anaesthetic and your doctor may well do it himself. Alternatively, he may refer you to a clinic. Either way, clipping the frenulum usually sorts the problem immediately and you will be encouraged to put your baby to the breast straight away. This stops any minor bleeding that may occur, as well as providing comfort for your baby.

Note: I see many mothers who have been told that their baby has tongue-tie simply because he is having latching problems. Most of these babies show none of the above symptoms and are able to latch on easily as soon as I show them how to do it properly.

And occasionally I will also come across a baby with extremely severe tongue-tie that has not been noticed either by the midwives or by the paediatrician who did the routine checks on the baby in hospital. If *you* think your baby has tongue-tie, do not assume that you must be wrong because no one else has picked up on it. Consult a doctor.

White nipple

This is a really painful condition (similar to Raynaud's syndrome) that may be associated with circulatory problems. When the baby feeds, the blood drains from the nipple causing intense pain and blanching of the nipple. Poor attachment of the baby to the breast and feeding in a cold room will often be the trigger for this.

Remedies that may help:

- Feed in a warmer room.
- Cover your breasts to keep them as warm as possible.
- Drinking tea before the feed may help dilate the blood vessels.
- Make sure your baby is latching on correctly (see page 29).

In severe cases your GP might prescribe the drug Nifedipine, which is often helpful in improving circulation. However, as this will pass into the breast milk and may affect the baby, you will need to discuss with your doctor whether it is advisable to try it.

Cranial osteopathy

There is growing interest in using osteopathy to treat babies who are suffering from a wide variety of problems ranging from colic to feeding or sleeping difficulties. In fact, many osteopaths believe that it would be beneficial to *all* babies to be given a routine check by an osteopath as soon as possible after the birth to 'iron out' any minor misalignments of the head or spine.

When I refer a baby to an osteopath, the mother will often report back that she has a 'new baby' who is now feeding or sleeping in a totally different way, and calm has now descended upon the household. Other mothers will say that it took several sessions before there was any real change but most of these also felt that it was well worth seeing an osteopath and that their baby had definitely benefited from the treatment.

What is cranial osteopathy?

Contrary to public misconception, a cranial osteopath will actually treat the whole body (not just the head) and the benefit to the baby is often immediate. The treatment is usually totally painless and involves very gentle manipulations of the skull and other parts of the body. This helps to release areas of stress and re-balance the whole body, not just the area that was worked upon.

The number of sessions required by your baby will depend upon the severity of his symptoms and your osteopath will usually be able to assess this at the first visit. Some babies only require one session.

What conditions may be helped by osteopathy?

- A crying, irritable baby who rarely settles well in between feeds, even though all his needs appear to have been met. He may be jumpy and react badly to loud noises. He may need to be held and cuddled a lot as he is unable to relax and go to sleep on his own.
- A baby who is having problems latching on to the breast and/or is failing to suck properly, even though you are using the correct technique to help him. He may chew rather than suck on your nipples, making you sore and preventing him from being able to 'milk' your breast efficiently. He may also feed noticeably better on one breast than the other, indicating that he is more uncomfortable on one particular side.
- A baby who rejects the breast in favour of the bottle, even though he appears to latch on easily and you have plenty of milk with a good flow. This baby will usually want a top-up bottle, regardless of how long he spends on the breast.
- A baby who feeds as badly from the bottle as he does from the breast. This baby will usually appear to have a poor sucking reflex and may take up to an hour to feed from a bottle, even using a teat with a fast flow. He may also feed noisily and messily and, in doing so, may suffer a lot with wind.

- A baby suffering from colic.
- A 'sicky' baby who regularly possets more than is usual.
- A baby who seems to need to do a lot of 'comfort sucking' either on the breast or a dummy.
- A baby with marked asymmetry of the head that persists long after the birth.

Although I am a fan of osteopathy for babies, I do still prefer to rule out normal reasons for the baby's symptoms before suggesting a mother consults an osteopath. This is because many babies will improve simply by changing the way the mother feeds or handles them. It is also important to rule out medical conditions (such as reflux) before going down the road of alternative treatments for your baby. If he has any of the above symptoms, I do recommend that you consult your doctor and/or a breast-feeding specialist as your first port of call. If they can't help, you may then find that an osteopath proves to be worth his weight in gold!

Starting solids

As this is essentially a breast-feeding book, I am not going to go into great detail about the whole business of giving solids (there are plenty of books devoted to this subject) but I do want to discuss *when* you should start. This is because mothers are generally given very 'politically correct' and inflexible advice on the subject, with no allowance being made for the fact that all babies are different and have different needs.

Back in the eighties, when my children were born, it was common practice to introduce solids at around three months and some particularly large and hungry babies were even given solids earlier than this. Then concerns were raised that solids given this early could cause long-term health problems and, as a result, mothers were told that they should not introduce solids until four months. Now, only a few years later, the World Health Organisation (WHO) recommends that babies should be exclusively breast-fed for six months and no solid food should be given before this time.

This is all very well in principle, but the reality is that many babies simply cannot wait this long and will become increasingly unhappy and unsettled if they are denied the comfort and calories of solid food. I have spoken to many doctors, paediatricians, etc., on the subject and, while many of them are aware that six months is an unrealistic target for quite a few babies, they are not prepared to put their head above the parapet and say so in public. I can understand their reluctance to do so, but nonetheless I think it is unfair on modern parents to be told to delay solids until six months simply to comply with government guidelines.

So, with this in mind, I would like to explain how you will know when *your* baby needs to start on solids and also to explain which foods are safe to give your baby.

First of all, I would agree that weaning *should* be delayed until six months whenever possible and would urge mothers only to introduce solid food before this time if your baby really cannot survive happily on milk alone.

Your baby probably needs solids if some or all of the following applies:

- He is at least four months old and weighs over 6 kg (13 lbs) (*he must fulfil this criteria before any of the following can be applied*).
- He is being offered as much milk as he will take at every feed, but is clearly getting hungry long before the next feed is due. If you are breast-feeding, you may need to offer a top-up and express after a few feeds in order to check that you are providing enough milk.
- He was down to four or five feeds a day, but is now demanding extra feeds.
- He was sleeping right through the night, but is now starting to wake again during the night, or earlier in the morning.
- He was *starting* to sleep longer at night, but is now waking more frequently than ever.
- He is chewing on his hands and generally looking dissatisfied after feeds.

If your baby is continually showing the above signs, you can gradually introduce some solid food into his diet, but make sure that you stick to simple and non-allergy forming foods until your baby reaches six months. The standard starting foods are baby rice (obtainable from chemists, etc.) along with puréed fruit and vegetables. You can also give any commercial baby foods that are marketed as being suitable for the age of your baby. By doing this, early weaning should have no adverse effect on his health.

It is also important to realise that solids should be offered in *addition* to your baby's usual amount of milk and should not be given as a replacement. You should therefore cut back or even stop giving solids altogether if your baby starts reducing his milk intake or shows signs of being less hungry. In other words, you should experiment to see how much food your baby needs and adjust accordingly.

Note: I do recommend that you buy a book on the subject of weaning that will give you much more comprehensive information on suitable foods and how to prepare and serve them. The information given here is only intended to be a guideline as to when to introduce solids.

How to get your baby to sleep through the night

How quickly a baby will start sleeping through the night is generally down to luck (rather than brilliant parenting!) but you can usually hope that your baby might start going longer at night from about six weeks. Some do it earlier than this and others quite a lot later, but in general a baby will gradually reduce night feeds when he is physically ready to do so, without any active measures being taken by you.

This is in the natural scheme of things and will normally happen provided your baby is getting plenty of milk during the day and that he has no physical problem (e.g. colic) that will disrupt his sleep.

A baby who has established a good feeding pattern consisting of regular feeds and plenty of sleep in between will almost always sleep better at night than a baby who is being fed totally 'on demand' without any attempt being made to establish a routine. Thus, a baby who is feeding three to four-hourly will usually sleep through the night sooner than a baby who is 'snacking' every hour or so and cat-napping throughout the day. Remember this – a relaxed, well-fed baby will sleep longer and better than a tense, over-tired baby.

With this in mind you should:

● Ensure that your milk supply is adequate so your baby always gets the amount of milk he needs.
● Try to space out feeds and organise your day so your baby is allowed to sleep in peace.
● Establish a routine whereby he is bathed, fed and settled quietly at a similar time each evening.
● Learn to recognise your baby's signals so you put him down to

sleep at exactly the right moment. If you put him down too early he won't be ready to drift off to sleep; if you leave it even a few minutes too late he will be over-tired and will be equally unable to settle

- Put him in a quiet room to sleep in the evening.
- Distinguish between night and day by feeding your baby at night with the lights dimmed.
- Make sure that he is not getting cold at night – you may need to start using a sleeping bag during the winter months if he is coming out from under his blankets.
- Decide whether you want to wake him for a 10pm feed (see page 86) or let him sleep through.

If you follow all the above advice, you will be fairly unlucky if your baby does not respond by sleeping well at night as soon as he is able to do so. Unfortunately some babies will inevitably be slower than others to sleep through for various medical reasons. For example, a premature baby will need night feeds for a lot longer than a full-term baby, and a baby suffering from reflux will only sleep through when successful treatment enables him to take larger feeds during the day.

There will also be a small number of babies who continue to wake at night for no obvious reason and you may just have to accept this as one of the trials and tribulations of parenthood. I do not believe that you should try to force a baby to sleep through the night until he is six months' old, at which point you could try various solutions that are on offer in many other baby books – I do not plan to go into any more detail myself as this is really a breast-feeding book, rather than a full child-care manual.

Note: My favourite book is *Toddler Taming* by Dr Christopher Green. He offers fantastic advice on all aspects of baby and child care and has an excellent section on sleep problems. And for those who would like to follow a more routine-based, step-by-step guide to caring for their baby, Gina Ford's book *The New Contented Little Baby Book* has proved invaluable for many mothers.

Final note

I do hope that every mother who reads this book will find at least something that proves to be helpful. If it helps to prevent even one problem from developing, I will feel that it has been worth all the hours it has taken me to write it! I would, however, like to remind all mothers that even if this book did not help you to establish successful breast-feeding, you should still give it a try if you have another baby. Many mothers find it is totally different the second time and are able to breast-feed for months on end without experiencing any of the problems that they may have had with their first baby.

Good luck!

Useful information and contacts

My DVD: 'Breast-feeding without Tears'
available by mail order, tel: 0870 420 8162
On this two-hour DVD you will see me teaching an ante-natal class, and also showing mothers how to latch their baby on to the breast, how to wind, swaddle, etc.

Medela UK
Tel: 0161 776 0400
Medela sells a huge range of breast-feeding products through mail order. I particularly recommend their breast pumps and nipple shields. You can also rent breast pumps from them.

Ameda Lactaline
Tel: 01823 336 362
I recommend their double breast pump for purchase or hire.

Babylist
50 Sulivan Road
London SW6 3DX
Tel: 020 7371 5145
Babylist will give you independent, unbiased advice to help you choose all the baby equipment and nursery items you'll need for your new baby.

Night Nannies
3 Kempson Road
London SW6 4PX
Tel: 020 7731 6168
Fax: 020 7610 9767
The Night Nannies agency will supply a qualified nurse or nanny to look after your child between the hours of 9pm and 7am. She will not only care for your child but will also assist you in trying to guide your baby to sleep through the night.

Doula UK
PO Box 26678
London N14 4WB
Tel: 0871 433 3103
Will provide you with all the information you need about hiring a doula.

Index

afterpains, while breast-feeding 21
air in baby's tummy see wind;
    winding
alcohol 10, 12
allergies 95, 168–9
anal stenosis (tight anal sphincter
    muscle) 153, 175, 176
antibiotics 74, 120-1, 153–5

baby
    breathing while feeding 32
    falling asleep while feeding 44–5
    feeding problems 135–62,
        178–80
    'fussing' at the breast 130-1
    growth spurts 129
    infection affecting feeding 132
    mouth defect affecting feeding
        132
    not sucking efficiently 131–3
    overheating 38–9
    positioning for feeding 24–5,
        27–9
    premature 132
    refusing bottle 94–5, 98, 156–61
    rejection of one breast 44
    settling on your lap 139–41
    signs of getting enough milk 33–5
    sleeping through feeds 86
    suitable room temperature 65–6
    time between feeds 35
    too weak to suck 49, 51, 52–3
    unsettled 55–7, 137–41, 142,
        144–53

    upset by fast milk flow 123–4
    yellowish skin 135–7
'baby blues' 62
baby clinic 70
baby monitor 65
baby seat, sleeping in 65
birth, and first few days 47–59
birth weight 75, 76
blocked milk ducts 118–19
bonding with a difficult baby 147–8
bottle-feeding 5, 6, 7, 163–76
    and tooth decay 173
    bottle refusal by baby 94–5, 98,
        156–61
    breast-fed baby 49–51, 94–5
    top-up to check milk supply
        142–3
breast
    before and after feeding 33–4
    engorged 2, 55, 57, 92, 113–17
    how milk is produced 14–16
    inflammation in 119–21
    red and hot area 119–21
    size and milk production 14
    small lumps on 118–19
    taking baby off 31–2
    vascular engorgement 117–18
breast abscess 121–2
breast-feeding 13–21, 23–45
    before your milk comes in 55–7
    check with top-up bottles 142–3
    combined with bottles 49–51,
        54–5, 156–61
    deciding not to start 162

feeding positions 24–5, 27–9, 41–5, 72
feeding problems (baby) 135–62, 178–80
feeding problems (mother) 101–33
first 24 hours 47–51
first few days 55–7
flow too fast for baby 123–4
frequency and regularity 57–8
how long to continue 95–6
in special care baby unit 161–2
introducing a bottle 94–5
latching on 29–33, 48, 55, 102–7
learning the technique 1–3, 55–7
let-down reflex 17–18
missing feeds 86–7
night feeds 86–7
one breast or both 19–21
preparation 5–9
starting up 15–16
stopping 95–8, 107
supply and demand 16–17
twins 43–4, 54–5, 71–4
when mother is ill 133
when your milk comes in 57–9
breast milk
alternating with formula feeds 107
expressing milk 58–9, 73, 89–94, 106–7, 111–12, 114–15, 116, 122–3
foremilk and hindmilk 18–19
freezing surplus 59, 90
guide to daily requirement 77
how it is produced 14–16
how much baby has taken 33–5
not enough milk 2, 125–9
things which affect the taste 130–1
time taken to dry up 96–8, 162
too much milk 122–3
ways to increase supply 126–9
breast milk jaundice 137 see also jaundice
breast pads 6
breast pumps 7–8, 89–90, 91, 93, 106–7, 111
breast shells 7, 122
breast surgery and breast-feeding 74–5

Caesarean section 16, 45
car seat, sleeping in 65

case histories
baby not sucking efficiently 131–3
baby too weak to suck 52–3
breast-feeding and bottle-feeding 54–5
helping baby to latch on 51–2
incorrect positioning causes sore nipples 112
milk flow too fast 124
poor feeding, baby dehydrated 53–4
primary engorgement 116–17
reflux 152–3
Child Health Record 76
colic 85, 130, 138, 144–8, 175
colostrum 14–15, 49, 55–7
constipation (baby) 98, 153
cot death risk 44, 89, 39
safety for baby 62–3
cows' milk allergies 144, 169
cranial osteopathy for babies 44, 132, 178–80
crying baby 41, 51, 80, 81, 82 see also unsettled baby
cup feeding 49–51, 173

dehydration (baby) 49, 51, 53–4, 131, 143, 155–6
demand feeding 80–3
diarrhoea 144
diet during pregnancy 9–10
diet while breast-feeding 10-11, 12, 143–4
district midwives 69–70
Domperidone 129
doulas 69
drugs, and breast-feeding 74
dummies 85, 87–9, 166

eczema, and milk allergy 144
engorged breasts 2, 55, 57, 92, 113–17 see also vascular engorgement
evening colic/fretting 148 see also colic
expressing milk 58–9, 73, 89–94, 106–7, 111–12, 114–15, 116, 122–3

feeding
and weight gain 75–7

frequency of 78–80, 82–4
general advice 71–99
jaundiced baby 136–7
length of time taken 78–80
on demand 80–3
settling into a routine 84–6
strict four-hourly schedule 83–4
see also bottle-feeding; breast-
feeding
feeding/nursing chair 27
fluid intake while breast-feeding 12
fontanelle, signs of dehydration 155
food intolerance 143–4
formula feeds 169–73
formula milk 7
allergies 144, 168–9
alternating with breast-feeds 107
disagreeing with baby 98, 168–9
feeding too little 155
for hungry baby 77
how much to offer 172–3
types available 168–9

gastro-oesophageal reflux see
reflux
goats' milk for babies 169
GP, confidence in 176
grandmother, helping with new
baby 67
growth spurts, and milk supply 129

health visitor 70
help, for new mothers 61–2, 66–70
hiccups, in babies 38
home, help for new mothers 61–2,
66–70
hospital, coming home from 61–70
hunger, in unsettled baby 138, 139,
148
husband, helping with new baby
66–7
hygiene 73–4, 164–7

immunity and colostrum 15
intracranial trauma, affecting
sucking reflex 132
inverted nipples 101–2

jaundice in babies 53–4, 131,
135–7

lactose intolerance 144

lap method of getting baby to
sleep 139–41
latching on 14, 23, 24–5, 29–31,
51–2, 72
problems with 2, 3, 102–7, 131–3
let-down reflex 17–18, 24–5
lips, rash and/or swelling 144
'lying in' after the birth 61–2

mastitis 2, 55, 115, 116–17, 119–21
maternity bras 6
maternity nurses 67–9
milk see breast milk; formula milk
milk allergy 142, 144, 145
milk ducts, blocked 43, 118–19
milk intolerance 138, 142, 145, 175
Moses basket 65
mouth defect, affecting feeding 132

nappy changing 26–7
nappy rash 26
night feeds 86–7
nipple creams 6, 8–9
nipple shields 7, 17–18, 102,
105–6, 109–11, 114, 123–4
nipples
inverted 101–2
preparation for breast-feeding
8–9
sore 2, 3, 8–9, 43, 55–7, 107–13
white nipple 178
Nipplette, to help inverted nipples
101–2

overheating of baby 38–9
overtiredness, unsettled baby 138,
139

paracetamol 74
partner, helping with new baby
66–7
phototherapy, for jaundice 135–6
possetting 37
premature baby 132
primary engorgement 113–17 see
also engorged breasts

reflux 98, 130, 138, 142, 145,
148–53, 175, 176
rest, importance of 61–2, 71–2
room temperature, suitable for
baby 65–6

rooting reflex 30

settling the baby 34, 35–41 see
    also unsettled baby
sleeping
    helping baby to settle 34, 35–41
        see also unsettled baby
    night waking due to cold 66
    pattern 86–7
    position of baby 39
    routine 86–7
    through the night 182–3
    where the baby should sleep
        63–65
sleepy baby 47–8, 48–9, 51, 131,
    136–7, 155
solids, starting on 174, 180–2
sore nipples 2, 3, 8–9, 43, 55–7,
    107–13
special care baby unit, feeding in
    161–2
sterilising 165–7
    equipment 5, 6, 164, 167–8
stools, indication of health 143,
    144, 153
sucking reflex 29, 31, 33, 81, 85,
    87–9
swaddling 38–41, 139

teats 164–5
thrush 142, 153–5
tongue-tie (ankyloglossia) 132,
    177–8

tooth decay, from bottle feeding
    173
top-up bottles, to check milk
    supply 142–3
twins, breast-feeding 43–4, 54–5,
    71–4

unsettled baby 137–41, 142,
    144–53 see also crying baby
urine, health indications 155

vascular engorgement 117–18
visitors, and new babies 62
vomiting 144

water
    drinking enough when breast-
        feeding 12
    for baby to drink 78, 85
weaning 181
    from breast to bottle 96–8
    starting on solids 174, 180–2
weighing a baby 33, 76
weight gain 19, 70, 75–7
    excessive 173–4
    poor 141–3, 148–53, 174–5
white nipple 178
wind 17–18, 85, 130, 138, 139,
    144–5
winding 34, 35–8, 172
working mothers, breast-feeding
    99

Also available from Vermilion

BIRTH AND BEYOND

Written by one of the world's leading obstetricians, this extraordinary book takes a totally fresh look at what parenting means at the beginning of the 21st century. Addressing both parents, the book looks at all aspects of life, through the nine months of pregnancy and the following nine of the baby's life. It is both a practical handbook for pregnancy, birth and the early months of a new baby's life, and a stimulating exploration of this period of enormous transition. Taking a holistic approach, it advocates integrated health care, i.e. both conventional and complementary therapies, and, with its exhaustive medical content, including a 160-page A-Z section, also acts as a superb source of reference.

Also available from Vermilion

NEW TODDLER TAMING
A parents' guide to the first four years

Dr Christopher Green

Revised and updated for the twenty-first century, *New Toddler Taming* offers friendly, practical advice for a new generation of parents with children at the challenging stage of toddlerdom, including:

- sleep solutions that really work
- successful potty training
- discipline – how to make life easier for yourself
- being a working parent
- the very latest of healthy eating

And much more!

Also available from Vermilion

YOU AND YOUR NEW BABY

Christine and Peter Hill

You and Your New Baby is a survival guide for new parents, helping them to adjust to life in the first few months after their baby is born. The authors take over from where other pregnancy books stop and before baby books begin. They provide a vast amount of practical and down-to-earth guidance on:

- what to expect in hospital and afterwards at home
- how to cope with persistent crying
- looking after yourself as well as your baby
- when and when not to return to work.

Drawing on the experiences of over 3000 mothers - and fathers - with new babies, and now fully updated, this authoritatative guide is both reassuring and fun to read.

ALSO AVAILABLE FROM VERMILION

☐	Birth and Beyond	9780091856946	£20.00
☐	New Toddler Taming	9780091875282	£12.99
☐	You and Your New Baby	9780091817121	£8.99

FREE POST AND PACKING
Overseas customers allow £2.00 per paperback

ORDER:

By phone: 01624 677237

By post: Random House Books
c/o Bookpost
PO Box 29
Douglas
Isle of Man, IM99 1BQ

By fax: 01624 670923

By email: bookshop@enterprise.net

Cheques (payable to Bookpost) and credit cards accepted

Prices and availability subject to change without notice.
Allow 28 days for delivery.
When placing your order, please mention if you do not wish to receive
any additional information

www.randomhouse.co.uk